A WOMAN'S BODY

A FULLY ILLUSTRATED GUIDE

Illustrations by Suzann Gage, L Ac, RNC,NP

Photographs by Sylvia Morales

FEMINIST HEALTH PRESS

A NOTE TO THE READER

The intention of this book is to assist women in learning more about well woman health care, self-examination, and well woman self care techniques. The health information shared in this book is not meant to replace the annual pap smear, or routine health or medical care. Rather, the information is intended to compliment the knowledge and expertise of health care providers, and to enable women to become more informed consumers in partnership with their health care practitioners. Advanced self-help techniques presented here, such as menstrual extraction, are not intended for use outside advanced self-help clinics. These techniques are used by women in advanced self-help groups who are specially trained in self-help skills.

1995 Printing By

Feminist Health Press
8240 Santa Monica Boulevard
Los Angeles, California 90046
(213) 650-1508 Fax (213) 848-9402

ISBN 0-9629945-0-2 Pbk.

with permission of the Federation of Feminist Women's Health Centers

First published 1981 by Simon and Schuster
IBSN 0-671-41214-0
ISBN 0-671-41215-9 Pbk.
Designed by Eve Kirch
Cover design by Anne Winslow

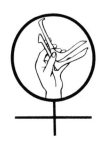

A NEW VIEW OF

by the Federation of Feminist
Women's Health Centers

DEDICATION

Over the past five years, while researching and writing this book or working at Feminist Women's Health Centers, we constantly thought of the women for whom this book was written. We dedicate this book to our mothers, daughters, sisters, lovers and friends . . .

Adele, Aggie Mae, Agnes, Alana, Albina, Alexia, Alicia, Alissa, Amber, Ana, Andrea, Angela, Ann, Anna, Anne, Annie, Arlene, Athena, Audrey, Azalea, Barbara, Becky, Bertye, Betty, Beverly, Birdie Faye, Bodil, Carmen, Carol, Carole, Caroline, Carolyn, Cathy, Cassidy, Cecilia, Chari, Chris, Collange, Connie, Conny, Cynthia, Daryl, Dolly, Dolores, Doreen, Dorothy, Dorrit, Dottie, Easter Mae, Ede, Elaine, Ele, Elizabeth, Ellen, Ellie, Emily, Enedina, Erin, Esther, Eurtie, Evelyn, Felicia, Fran, Frances, Gemma, Ginger, Ginny, Gladys, Gloria, Grace, Haikila, Heidi, Helen, Henrietta, Irene, Janessa, Jean, Jeanne, Jeannette, Jennifer, Jenny, Jill, Jo, Joan, Joanne, Jody, Josann, Joy, Joyce, Judy, Julia, June, Karen, Katherine, Khrista, Kirsten, Kyla, Laura, Lauren, Laurie, Lenore, Leslie, Lillian, Lindsay, Lois, Lois Jeanne, Lori, Lorna, Lorraine, Lou, Lupe, Lydia, Lynn, Mal, Margaret, Margie, Margo, Maria Elena, Marie, Marina, Marion, Marla, Martha, Mary, Mary Jo, Mary Lou, Meg, Melba, Melodie, Mercedes, Merissa, Merrie, Micaela, Mildred, Millie, Missy, Molly, Muriel, Mya, Myrna, Nancy, Natasha, Nell, Nola, Pam, Pamela, Pat, Paulina, Peggy, Phaedra, Phoebe, Phyllis, Regina, Rosa, Rose, Rosemary, Roxanne, Ruth, Sally, Sandra, Sara, Sarah, Shannon, Sharon, Sharron, Shatiris, Sheila, Shelby, Sherita, Sophie, Suzanne, Sylvia, Tamar, Tami, Teri, Terry, Thelma, Theresa, Toni, Torrie, Valerie, Velma, Verda, Vicki, Virginia, Zenovia.

ILLUSTRATIONS: Suzann Gage

GENERAL EDITOR: Carol Downer

EDITOR: Rebecca Chalker

COORDINATOR: Sandra Sullaway

CONTRIBUTORS: Carol Downer
Francie Hornstein
Lorraine Rothman
Jennifer Burgess
Sherry Schiffer
Shelley Farber
Dido Hasper
Lynn Heidelberg
Ginny Cassidy-Brinn
Marcia Kerwit
Janet Cuddihy
Kathleen Hodge
Suzann Gage
Thora DeLey
Carol Koury

PHOTOGRAPHS: Sylvia Morales

CONTENTS

List of Illustrations   8

Acknowledgments   11

Preface   13

ONE   The Grassroots of Self-Help   17

TWO   Self-Examination   21

THREE   The Clitoris: A Feminist Perspective   33

FOUR   A Woman's Reproductive Anatomy   59

FIVE   A Well-Woman Exam   79

SIX   Universal Health Problems of Women   87

SEVEN   Birth Control   105

EIGHT   Menstrual Extraction   121

NINE   Feminist Abortion Care   129

TEN   Serious Health Problems: Surgery   137

ELEVEN   A Self-Help Clinic   153

Glossary   155

Appendix: Women's Health Projects   164

Bibliography   168

Index   171

Photo section follows page 128

LIST OF ILLUSTRATIONS

Illus. no.		Page
2-1	A Woman Inserting a Speculum	22
2-2	A Woman Opening a Speculum	23
2-3	A View of the Cervix in a Mirror	24
2-4	Plastic Vaginal Speculums	25
2-5	A Woman Doing Self-Examination with a Medium Speculum (Incorrect Size)	26
2-6	A Woman Doing Self-Examination with a Long Speculum (Correct Size)	26
2-7	A Woman's-Eye View of Breast Self-Examination	27
2-8	A Woman Feeling Her Ribs Through Her Breast	27
2-9	A Woman Looking in a Mirror	28
2-10	A Woman Raising Her Arms While Looking in a Mirror	28
2-11	Squeezing the Nipple	28
2-12	A Woman Feeling the Upper Part of Her Breast	29
2-13	A Woman Feeling Her Nipple	29
2-14	A Woman Feeling Her Armpit	29
2-15	A Woman Lying Down with a Pillow Under Her Shoulder	30
2-16	A Woman Feeling the Upper Part of Her Breast While Lying Down	30
2-17	A Woman Feeling Her Nipple While Lying Down	30
2-18	A Woman Feeling Her Armpit While Lying Down	30
2-19	A Woman Lying on Her Back Feeling a Folded Breast Gland	31
2-20	A Woman With Stretch Marks on Her Breasts	31
3-1	An Outer View of the Clitoris	34
3-2	The Glans of the Clitoris	35
3-3	A Woman Doing Self-Examination of the Clitoris by Rolling the Shaft	36
3-4	A Woman Doing Self-Examination of the Clitoris by Squeezing the Glans	36
3-5	The Outer Anatomy of the Clitoris	37
3-6	The Muscles of the Clitoris	38
3-7	The Erectile Tissue of the Clitoris	39
3-8	The Pelvic Muscles (without the Clitoris)	40
3-9	A Cross Section of the Clitoris	41
3-10	A Detailed View of the Clitoris in the Pelvis	42
3-11	Inset: The Pelvic Bones	42
3-12	A Detailed View of the Clitoris Showing the Urethral Sponge	43
3-13	Self-Examination of the Urethral Sponge	44
3-14	Self-Examination of the Perineal Sponge	45
3-15	The Nerves of the Clitoris	46
3-16	A Side View of the Clitoris: Compared to the Penis	48
3-17	A Side View of the Penis: Compared to the Clitoris	49
3-18	An Outer View of the Nonerect Clitoris	50
3-19	An Inner View of the Nonerect Clitoris	50
3-20	An Outer View of the Clitoris During the Excitement Phase	51
3-21	An Inner View of the Clitoris During the Excitement Phase	51
3-22	An Outer View of the Clitoris During the Plateau Phase	51
3-23	An Inner View of the Clitoris During the Plateau Phase	51

3-24	An Outer View of the Clitoris During the Orgasm Phase	52
3-25	An Inner View of the Clitoris During the Orgasm Phase	52
3-26	The Clitoral Muscles During the Orgasm Phase	52
3-27	The Pelvic Muscles During the Orgasm Phase	52
3-28	An Outer View of the Clitoris During the Resolution Phase	53
3-29	An Inner View of the Clitoris During the Resolution Phase	53
3-30	Female Ejaculation	54
3-31	The Uterus During Sexual Arousal	55
3-32	A Cross Section of the Nonerect Clitoris	56
3-33	A Cross Section of the Clitoris During Sexual Arousal	57
4-1	A Seated Woman with Her Uterus Visible	58
4-2	An Inner View of a Woman's Breast	60
4-2A	Inset: A Breast Gland	61
4-3	The Secretions of the Vulva, Clitoris and Vagina	63
4-4	The Uterus in the Pelvis, Left Side	64
4-5	The Uterus in the Pelvis, ¾ Turn to the Right	64
4-6	The Uterus in the Pelvis, Front View	64
4-7	The Uterus in the Pelvis, ¾ Turn to the Left	64
4-8	The Uterus in the Pelvis, Right Side	64
4-9	A View of the Uterus, Intestines and Bladder	65
4-10	A View of the Uterus and Bladder with the Intestines Not Shown	66
4-11	A View of the Uterus with the Intestines and Bladder Not Shown	67
4-12	A Woman with a Tipped-Up Uterus Doing Self-Examination	68
4-13	A Woman with a Midline Uterus Doing Self-Examination	68
4-14	A Woman with a Tipped-Back Uterus Doing Self-Examination	69
4-15	The Glands Which Secrete Hormones: The Endocrine Glands	70
4-16	The Ovary with Primary Follicles	72
4-17	The Ovary with Secondary Follicles	72
4-18	The Ovary with Tertiary Follicle	73
4-19	The Ovary at the Moment of Ovulation	73
4-20	The Opening of the Egg Tubes Above the Ovary	73
4-21	The Ovary with the Corpus Luteum (Yellow Body) After Ovulation	73
4-22	The Egg Tube Contracting	74
4-23	The Lining of the Uterus	75
5-1	A Health worker Doing a Uterine Size Check	78
5-2	Pap Smear: Cells Being Taken from the Face of the Cervix	80
5-3	Pap Smear: Cells Being Taken from the Vagina	80
5-4	Pap Smear: Cells Being Taken from the Opening of the Cervix	80
5-5	Pap Smear: Spraying Preservative on the Pap Smear Slide	81
5-6	Trichomonas and Yeast Seen Through a Microscope	82
5-7	The Urine Pregnancy Test	83
5-8	The Techniques of Cervical Cauterization	84
5-9	A Gonorrhea Culture	85
5-10	Donor Insemination	85
6-1	A Woman Feeling a Breast Cyst	86
6-2	Genital Warts	88
6-3	The Vulvovaginal Glands	88
6-4	A Vulvovaginal Gland Cyst	88
6-5	Discharge from an Overgrowth of Yeast and from Trichomonas	89
6-6	Sucking Air: A Technique to Aid in the Application of Vaginal Remedies	90
6-7	A Group of Active Herpes Blisters	91
6-8	The Squamocolumnar Junction	92
6-9	An Infection of the Cervical Canal	93
6-10	Cysts on the Cervix	94
6-11	Uterine Fibroids and Cervical Polyps	95
6-12	A Uterine Size Check for Fibroids	96
6-13	A Relaxation Technique to Relieve Menstrual Cramps	97
6-14	First Step of the Cobra Exercise to Relieve Menstrual Cramps	98
6-15	Second Step of the Cobra Exercise	98
6-16	Third Step of the Cobra Exercise	98
6-17	Direct Uterine Massage to Relieve Menstrual Cramps	99
6-18	Lower Back Massage to Relieve Menstrual Cramps	99
6-19	First Step of the Bow Exercise to Relieve Menstrual Cramps	99
6-20	Second Step of the Bow Exercise	99
6-21	Direct Pressure Point Massage to Relieve Menstrual Cramps	100
6-22	*Shiatsu* Massage to Relieve Menstrual Cramps	100
6-23	A View of the Urinary Tract	101
6-24	Devices to Absorb or Catch Menstrual Flow	103
7-1	A Basal Body Temperature Chart	107
7-2	The Effects of Self-Observation as Birth Control	108
7-3	The Effects of Local Methods as Birth Control	108
7-4	The Effects of IUDs as Birth Control	109
7-5	The Effects of the Pill as Birth Control	109
7-6	A Cross Section of the Cervix with Fertile Mucus	110
7-6A	Inset: The Structure of Fertile Mucus	110

7-6B   Inset: An Endocervical Gland with
    Fertile Mucus   110
7-7   A Cross Section of the Cervix with
    Nonfertile Mucus   111
7-7A   Inset: The Structure of Nonfertile Mucus   111
7-7B   Inset: An Endocervical Gland with
    Nonfertile Mucus   111
7-8   How to Insert a Diaphragm   112
7-9   How to Check a Diaphragm   113
7-10   How to Remove a Diaphragm   113
7-11   Correctly and Incorrectly Fit Diaphragms   114
7-12   The Cervical Cap   114
7-13   A Condom on an Erect Penis   115
7-14   Step One of IUD Insertion   116
7-15   Step Two of IUD Insertion   117
7-16   An IUD Inserted   118
8-1   Menstrual Extraction Equipment   122
8-2   A Woman Having a Uterine Size Check
    Before Menstrual Extraction   123
8-3   A Woman Inserting Her Speculum   124
8-4   The Woman who is Having the
    Extraction Pumping the Del-Em   124
8-5   A Self-Helper Inserting the Cannula   125
8-6   A Woman Holding the Cannula with
    O-Ring Forceps   126
8-7   The Cannula Inserted into the Uterus   126
8-8   Chorionic Villi in a Glass   127
9-1   A Woman Having an Early Suction
    Abortion   130
9-2   An Early Suction Abortion   132
9-3   An Early Suction Abortion Completed   133
9-4   A Laminaria Stick   134
9-5   Dilators of Different Sizes   134
9-6   A Saline Abortion   135
10-1   A View of a Healthy Woman's Breasts   136
10-2   Different Parts of the Breasts Which May
    Be Removed During Surgery   140

10-3   Aspiration of a Breast Cyst   140
10-4   Lumpectomy: Tissue Affected by
    Removal of a Lump   141
10-5   Segmental Mastectomy: Tissue Affected
    by Removal of a Lump and
    Surrounding Tissue   141
10-6   Simple Mastectomy: Tissue Affected by
    Removal of Breast Tissue Down to the
    Muscles   142
10-7   Modified Radical Mastectomy: Tissue
    Affected by Removal of the Breast and
    Lymph Nodes   142
10-8   Radical Mastectomy: Tissue Affected by
    Removal of the Breast, Lymph Nodes
    and Muscles   143
10-9   A Scar from a Radical Mastectomy   143
10-10   Clipping the Egg Tubes for Sterilization   144
10-11   The Dilation for a D and C   145
10-12   Curetting, or Scraping Away the Uterine
    Lining During a D and C   146
10-13   Step One in Opening the Abdominal
    Wall for Pelvic Surgery   147
10-14   Step Two in Opening the Abdominal
    Wall   147
10-15   The Uterus Before a Hysterectomy
    (Bladder is Not Shown)   148
10-16   The Pelvic Area After a Simple
    Hysterectomy   149
10-17   The Pelvic Area After a Radical
    Hysterectomy   149
10-18   First Step of a Conization   150
10-19   Second Step of a Conization   150
10-20   A Punch Biopsy   150
10-21   The Vas Deferens After a Vasectomy   151
11-1   A Self-Help Group   152

ACKNOWLEDGMENTS

Many women laid the groundwork which ultimately resulted in this book. In 1975, en route to New York City to find a publisher and an agent, we interviewed and photographed many health activists. We thank those women who took the time to answer our questions, took us into their homes and posed for photographs for a book that was to go through many changes before it was finally published. Ann Morehead, then from the Oakland Feminist Women's Health Center, was a member of the group originally delegated to work on the book, which we have called the Book Team. We thank her, Laura Brown and Debra Law, also from the Oakland Feminist Women's Health Center, for their participation in those early efforts.

We thank the feminist authors and editors who encouraged us and shared their experiences with agents and publishers. In New York, Kirsten Grimstad and Susan Rennie met with us and Robin Morgan set up appointments for us with several feminist editors, all of whom were helpful, especially Edite Kroll. In Boston, we met with Judy Norsigian and Norma Swenson of the Boston Women's Health Book Collective who accompanied us to see several editors.

The various drafts of the manuscript have been read by many women at the various health centers and throughout the Women's Health Movement. We thank these women for their time and valuable suggestions. We are especially appreciative of the many hours that the women of the Boston Women's Health Book Collective devoted to a critical reading of the final manuscript. Their contribution resulted in many valuable improvements.

Many people shared the results of their work with us, answering questions, locating references and commenting on what we had written. We would like to thank Linda Bennett and Tonya Brooks of the Association for Childbirth at Home International; Sarah Berndt and the New Hampshire Feminist Health Center; Debra Bing of the Julius Schmid Laboratories; Christine Brim of the National Abortion Rights Action League; Milos Chvapil, MD, of the University of Arizona; Cathy Courtney of the Detroit Health Department; Laura Cristal of Responsible Parenthood, San Diego, California; Catherine Dirk; Christopher Dotson, MD; Ginny Evans; Caleb Finch, MD, and Maureen Leyva of the University of Southern California; Debbie Freeman of the Westside Women's Clinic, Santa Monica, California; Barbara Haas; Judith Hall, MD; Robert Hatcher, MD, of Emory University School of Medicine; Hubert Hemsley, MD, of the Bethune Medical Center, Compton, California; Calvin Hobel, MD, of Harbor General Hospital, Los Angeles; Edward Keefe, MD; AnnaKria King; Diana Lane of the University of California at Fullerton Medical Library; Helen Marieskind, editor of *Women and Health;* Henry Maso; Robert Mendelsohn, MD; Darrel Meyes; William Moss, MD; Howard Ory, MD, Diana Pettiti, MD, and George Stroh of the Center for Disease Control; Peter Philander and William Southern, MD, of the Upjohn Company; Bernard Rosenfeld, MD; Julius Roth; Gordon Rubin; Barbara Seaman; Christopher Tietze, MD, of the Population Council; Jean Trueblood of Planned Parenthood, Los Angeles; Gloria Wahlquist; Barbara Waldford; and Kay Weiss of the Stanford Research Institute.

We thank Joanne Tanihara for her excellent typing on an early manuscript; the women at HealthRight for the loan of very hard-to-find reference material; Jane Molson for her assistance to the Book Team; Judy Myers Suchey, Ph.D. for the loan of the model of a woman's pelvis; Alicia Castorena for skillfully assisting the photographer; Ruth Peskin for the use of her darkroom and equipment; Karen Grant for participating in the hormone study; Jan Haaken for her information shared and work on the hormone study; Jack Sandweis for his support; Yanella Friedman, Pat Maginnis and Lana Phelan for sharing their experiences with us; Gabrielle Karsten for the discussions her comments generated; and Sheryl Ruzek, Jackie Stefko, Lolly and Jeanne Hirsch, Jackie McMillan, Susan Clark, Judy Koretsky and Jean-Philippe Benaim for their encouragement and interest; Claudine Serre, whose annual visits were a source of inspiration and a contribution to our perspective.

We want to especially acknowledge Marion Banzhaf and Rebecca Pierson for their work on the list of women's health projects and Chris Cleary, Nancy Walker and Lynn Walker for photographing the sexual response cycle.

We are indebted to Hugh Meddings, the loan officer at Security Pacific National Bank, who made it possible by extending our loan more than once for us to continue our work.

There are a number of people whose contributions were central to writing this book. In addition to supporting the work of the health centers during the time this book was written, they thoughtfully read and commented on portions of the manuscript. Vicki Jones, Willard Cates, MD, and David Grimes, MD, of the Center for Disease Control in Atlanta, Georgia, provided information, assistance and shared their research with us. Jane Patterson, MD, was always available to answer our questions and read an earlier manuscript for medical correctness. Theodora Wells, feminist writer who specializes in management consultation, edited portions of the manuscript at key times in its evolution. Malcolm Jones, a self-helper from Martha's Vineyard, and his family generously donated to this project. Alvin H. Rothman, professor of biology at California State University at Fullerton, provided invaluable assistance. Along with reviewing the manuscript's technical information, Al worked with four of us, "the hormone team," over a period of months, informally lecturing, until we were able to grasp the highly complex information about hormones. Numerous donations to a book fund established in memory of Joy Maso were gratefully received.

The Book Team worked at the Downer house for most of the book's writing. We are most grateful to Frank Downer, Angela Downer, Frankie Downer and David Brown for allowing us to take over most of their home as well as their telephone.

Dorrit Thomsen supplied an additional photo for the color insert.

We especially want to thank Susan Bolotin, our editor at Simon and Schuster, who urged us to do this book and then assisted us in adapting our ideas to this format. We also want to thank Roz Siegel for her guidance and consideration in helping us tie up the loose ends. And we thank Claire Smith, our agent, who since the beginning has encouraged us and given us nothing but the soundest counsel.

Finally, we want to express our thanks to those women who worked at the Feminist Women's Health Centers while the book was being written. We especially want to thank Marilyn Skerbeck, Ellen Peskin and Roberta Maso of the Los Angeles Feminist Women's Health Center who worked in the clinic and gave direction to the health centers while we were off writing the book. They worked 60 hours and more, week after week, often at partial salary so work on the book could continue. We also want to acknowledge the contribution of other women in Los Angeles: Teri Albright, Edith Berg, Camilla Cracchiolo, Ana Luisa Garcia-Ponce, Gail Goldstein, Sara Grusky, Linda Hart, Margo Miller, Wendy Radatz, Claudia Sperber, Lisa Tackley and Dorrit Thomsen. Certain women of the Chico Health Center deserve particular acknowledgment: Jeannie Clayton, Chris Cleary, Maeve Dunn, Hillary Emmer, Shauna Heckert, Vicki Keeran, Delores Nolan, Maureen Pierce and Lisa Todd. In Orange County, we want to thank Deborah Lazaldi, Eileen Schnitger, Eleanor Snow, Lynn Walker and Nancy Walker; and in San Diego, Sol Barreto, Mary Ann Bennett, Karen Black, Ann Collins, Julie Hocking, Hortense McGinnis, Cindy Pearson and Debi Stuart-Smalley. In addition, we want to acknowledge the women in Atlanta, Georgia: Susan Byers, Janet Callum, Kathryn Davis, Mary Lynn Hemphill, Lynne Randall and Lynn Thogerson; and in Tallahassee, Florida: Marion Banzhaf, Linda Curtis, Risa Denenberg, Susan Griffin, Dawn Husky and Rebecca Pierson.

The Book Team
September, 1980

PREFACE

by Jane Patterson, M.D.

The first time I heard about self-help clinics was a few years ago when NBC News asked me for my opinion of them. I have been in practice since 1968 as an obstetrician and gynecologist and knowing that most women are abysmally ignorant of their bodies, I found the concept appealing. But before I could make a statement, I first had to find out what self-help clinics were. Told that the Feminist Women's Health Center (FWHC) would be taking part in the proposed broadcast, I went to their Los Angeles clinic, the first to be opened.

The women there, I observed, share what they have learned in the course of helping themselves. The clinic encourages the use of safe methods of contraception and stresses the necessity for continued and women-controlled research into the efficacy of all methods of contraception.

Impressed by the FWHC's emphasis on knowledge and on safety, I agreed to participate in the NBC program, especially since I was so angry at having prescribed IUDs and sequential birth control pills which had been represented to me as safe. I thought I was benefiting my patients, only to find out—through the lay media, not from professional sources—that I had exposed women entrusted to my care to the risk of malignancy and death.

Since my introduction to the FWHC, I have learned a great deal more about the benefits of the self-help principle as it unfolds in the FWHC clinics.

In my practice I have learned how much more help I can give to a patient who can describe and discuss with me what is happening to her. We can talk together as equals, exchanging infomation, and it is a great relief to both of us that I can finally give up the Medical Deity role.

There is no reason why women shouldn't have as much information about their bodies as physicians do. Yet busy physicians cannot find time to educate patients adequately, so women still risk complications and even death because they are unable to find information that is kept behind locked doors. This book breaks down these barriers.

I think it was Talleyrand who said that war was too important to be left to the generals. I would like to suggest that the health of women is too important to be left to the medical establishment.

I am concerned about what government regulatory agencies are doing to help women, if they are doing anything. I am angry at women's being used as guinea pigs and sick of reading articles that take research data on rats and extrapolate them to women.

Among other areas, there is a need for women-controlled research of birth control methods: research on methods most advantageous to women is not being reported in the current literature. I am angry to read in my own medical journals the multiple, repetitious and contradictory articles on the complications of current contraceptives. And when I read, "We wish to express sincere appreciation to X drug company for funding this study," I wonder about the ethics of the research being described.

Even though I have been trained as a physician, I too, have experienced, as a woman, the euphoria that comes from knowing that we can now know, on our own, what to do for ourselves, and know what kind of health care we need. Where information is readily available to women about themselves, they can make informed choices regarding their own health and their own bodies.

As a physician, I have not been involved in writing this book—it has all been done by women no more trained in medicine than most of you readers.

It is high time for a book like this!

This book will help both women and their physicians to achieve a far higher quality of health care.

Here it is. Go to it!

Los Angeles
December, 1980

A NEW VIEW OF A WOMAN'S BODY

1 • The Grassroots of Self-Help

This book celebrates the diversity and uniqueness of women's bodies; at the same time, it joyously asserts our commonality. If a woman's body is otherwise healthy, her breasts are not too large or too small, she is not too fat or too thin, nor is she too hairy. Whether her cycles are short or long, whether she has children or not, whether she has sex with men or with women, this book seeks to address a variety of her health needs.

Our healthy secretions deserve to be understood in the same way that we comprehend any of our bodies' functions. This book acknowledges every woman's right to know how she experiences orgasm. It seeks to break down the barriers between women and to replace them with new ways of communication. It offers new concepts, including the use of inexpensive, safe home remedies, which make it possible to deal with many eternal health problems. And it encourages women to be more assertive health-care consumers.

Thousands of women who have done self-examination of the cervix and vagina in group settings called self-help clinics conceived these new concepts. Over the past decade, they have shared with us the knowledge that they have gained, which is in turn being shared with you in this book.

Suzann Gage's well-researched illustrations are designed to lift the veil of medical mystery from women's bodies and reveal truths that, though simple, have been hidden up to now. We believe that many of these illustrations are superior to any to be found in medical texts.

The First Self-Help Clinic

Our society is full of negative images of women's bodies. Billboards clutter the streets with blowups of scantily clad women selling liquor, cigarettes, records or vacations. Magazines with pictures of women lolling on couches in silk underwear, with their legs spread open, appear out of businessmen's briefcases on planes or trains. Rock 'n' roll albums rely heavily on depictions of violence toward women to sell their contents. Although the need for positive, helpful images of women seems urgent, magazine editors have been uninterested in printing photographs showing women readers how to learn more about their bodies through self-examination. Likewise, high school teachers and principals have repeatedly censored our ten-minute film showing self-examination of the vagina with a plastic speculum, thus denying young women one of the basic means of learning more about their reproductive and sexual organs. Women are given a very clear message: be sexually available, but do not look at, touch or understand your bodies.

The first self-help clinic arose out of these contradictions.

Although our group now has more of a mixed composition—single women, lesbians, women of color and very young women—in 1970, we were six white housewives who had 24 children among us, and a combined medical experience of over a hundred years. We organized a meeting held in Los Angeles on April 7, 1971, to devise strategies to change the abortion laws which prohibited us from controlling our own reproduction and, thus, our own lives. With other women who joined us, we spent the first half of the evening doing self-examination on a desk in an alcove. Then we sat in a circle on the floor and talked for the last half of the evening, discussing our health care and experiences with the medical profession, in an attempt to sift and sort out our common feelings. We explained to the group how much we could learn by doing self-examination and by conducting frank discussions. Together, we discovered how much our image of our bodies, particularly our genitals, improved after self-examination.

Self-Help on Tour

Through low-budget trips, financed primarily by donations, with food and lodging provided by our hosts, we spread the ideas of self-help throughout the Women's Liberation Movement. We spoke at campus women's centers, at chapter meetings of the National Organization for Women and at consciousness-raising sessions. We realized that if we received so many benefits from self-help, so must other women. Traveling provided us with an opportunity to meet them and to learn first hand what was going on outside our own communities.

Soon after our first cross-country trip, we were given the use of two rooms in the Los Angeles Women's Center for a phone, a desk and a table on which to demonstrate self-examination. Of the groups we met and the groups we organized, many went on from their weekly self-help clinic sessions to become more involved in women's health care. Some expanded their new understanding by reading medical texts and by working on solving some of the age-old problems plaguing many women. Through self-examination, we gained the knowledge to become aggressive medical consumers.

Some groups established a women's night at their local free clinics, or sent some members to school to become nurses, physicians or paraprofessionals.

We Became Health-Care Consumer Advocates

In addition to our weekly self-help clinics, our Los Angeles group started an abortion referral service. We received blocks of time at the hospital during which women could receive abortions from our handpicked physicians. We accompanied women and counseled them every step of the way, making sure they received nontraumatic abortions in a respectful atmosphere. This not only gave us a financial base upon which to open our health center, now called the Feminist Women's Health Center, in a large, two-story house, but it also gave us entry into hospitals where we could observe the medical profession at close range.

When we called ourselves "feminists" in 1971, we took a 19th-century term and dusted it off. Organizations such as the National Organization for Women (NOW) called themselves "women's rights groups," and loosely structured consciousness-raising groups and grassroots women's centers saw themselves as "women's liberation." Feminism denoted to us an organized fight against the patriarchy, not just getting a piece of the pie or causing social changes by creating alternative social structures. Currently most women who are involved in any of these approaches define themselves as feminists.

Self-Help Clinic's First Challenge

Of course, women flocking to our self-help clinic did not go unnoticed by the medical profession. In September of 1972, we were raided by the Department of Consumer Affairs of the State of California, the enforcement arm of the Board of Medical Examiners (BME). One doctor, three uniformed policemen and several plainclothes investigators confiscated four truckloads of equipment and supplies and later arrested two women, Carol Downer and Colleen Wilson, for practicing medicine without a license.

Based on the reports of an undercover agent, Wilson was charged with 11 counts; she pled guilty to one count of practicing medicine without a license—specifically, fitting a diaphragm. When Downer asked the BME doctor if he considered a mother's diagnosis of her child's measles to be practicing medicine without a license, he replied, "Well, we can't do anything about *that*."

The charge against Downer arose from the fact that she had inserted yogurt into the vagina of a Women's Center staff member. At the trial, which became known as "The Great Yogurt Conspiracy," she was found not guilty, using the defense that applying yogurt as a home remedy for an ordinary yeast condition is not practicing medicine. Her acquittal definitely established women's rights to learn more about their own bodies through self-examination.

The trial attracted national attention, and was covered in *Time, Newsweek* and the *New York Times.* Support from hundreds of women came in the form of donations and affidavits stating that they had used a speculum, and prominent women such as Gloria Steinem, Bella Abzug, Margaret Mead and Robin Morgan made public statements of support.

We Became Health Educators

Instead of stopping us, the medical profession had inadvertently given us a boost. We traveled even more widely and spoke at campuses and conferences about self-help. In 1972, we held a self-help conference in Iowa attended by women from across the U.S. and Canada, including Jeanne and Lolly Hirsch, feminists from Connecticut who started a magazine, *The Monthly Extract: an Irregular Periodical.* In 1973, Lorraine Rothman was invited by women in New Zealand to bring them the new ideas of self-help, and Carol Downer and Debra Law made a European tour.

After the Supreme Court decision that abortion in the first 12 weeks of pregancy was a matter to be decided by a woman and her physician, we and many other women's health groups were able to open our own abortion clinics. We refurbished a duplex on Crenshaw Boulevard near downtown Los Angeles that had been the Women's Center. The kitchen was our sterilizing room and the rooms in which we had been doing self-examination and abortion counseling became the exam rooms in which women received their abortions. We met the Health Department's regulations for clinical licensing, bargained with medical suppliers, bought malpractice insurance and trained physicians in better, less traumatic abortion techniques.

After we had developed participatory health care, many of our ideas were accepted and emulated by others. In our participatory clinics, women learn vaginal, cervical and breast self-examination, and receive their Pap smears, birth control pills or screening tests in a group. Now, most abortion facilities have counselors to give women step-by-step information about the abortion and to provide support as they go through the procedure. Many physicians now keep a mirror in the exam room to show women their cervixes during examinations. It has become fashionable for the medical profession to use terms similar to those we developed, such as "well-woman health care," "participatory clinic" and "women's heath-care specialist," to describe their programs.

We have been invited to prestigious professional gatherings, such as the conferences of the American Public Health Association and the American Psychological Association, to lecture on self-help and the treatment of women by the health establishment, and we are active in numerous national organizations, including the National Abortion Federation.

We Became a Federation

Women in other communities, inspired by self-help, traveled to the Los Angeles Health Center to learn how to run a women-controlled clinic. Women in the early self-help clinics established other Feminist Women's Health Centers in Santa Ana and Oakland, California. In 1973 and 1974, the California health centers offered a summer institute in which the skills of administering a business and of maintaining a group dedicated to social change were shared. Women came from all over the United States, Canada and Europe. Some of them shared our philosophy so closely that they started their own Feminist Women's Health Centers in Detroit, Michigan; Tallahassee, Florida; and Chico, California. Later, women in San Diego, California; Atlanta, Georgia; and Berlin, West Germany, also started health centers. The staffs of several of the health centers in the United States wanted to work very closely together and formed the Federation of Feminist Women's Health Centers, which now comprises the health centers in Santa Ana, Los Angeles, Chico, San Diego and Atlanta. Everywoman's Clinic in Concord, California, is an associate member.

During these same years, many women-controlled clinics were established, incorporating the ideas of self-help. All of the women who participated in these projects were a part of the growing women's movement. They worked together in a national network to focus on critical issues in women's health: reproductive rights, including abortion and safe birth control, home birth, women's right to respectful health care, sterilization abuse, medical experimentation on women and the right to informed consent, and on unnecessary and disfiguring surgery, especially mastectomy and hysterectomy. This national network of feminists became the Women's Health Movement. Today, there are 23 women-controlled abortion clinics and approximately 106 women's health projects in the United States.

There was one way that self-help could travel to more women than we could ever reach in years of plane trips, bus rides or cross-country car marathons: a *book.* In 1975, our decision to write our first book, *Women's Health in Women's Hands,* which is a large, heavily detailed health book, forced us into a new spurt of growth. As writers, we delved into the medical textbooks and mastered the complexities of endocrinology to the extent that we were able to critique the current ideas on hormone functions. The process of writing that book and this one has meant years of studying the medical literature, both scholarly and popular, reading feminist writings, extensive discussion and many sessions of self-examination. Much of our information and many of our ideas came from running our own women's clinics. We were fortunate, also, to have access to laboratory facilities and to have many friends in the healtn professions who shared their expertise and knowledge with us.

To write our first book, we waded through many textbooks and studies, among them Masters and Johnson's *Human Sexual Response,* which we found unnecessarily dense and abstruse. We looked at anatomical drawings and then looked at our own vulvas and clitorises to check Masters and Johnson's validity. In the process, we surprised ourselves by coming to some new conclusions about female sexual response that seem to us much more sensible and plausible than Masters and Johnson's. We realized while doing this research that we needed to redefine the clitoris. We discovered that it was not only the small shaft, glans and hood, but the muscles, blood vessels, nerves and other tissues that actively respond in sexual excitement. These new concepts are based on widely accepted facts; our contribution has been to organize these facts from a woman's point of view.

We Became Self-Help Researchers

Suzann Gage went through an arduous process in drawing the illustrations. She and a model would discuss the best way to portray a particular concept. The model, usually an experienced self-helper, would do vaginal self-examination and then Suzann would do a uterine size check to ascertain the size and location of the uterus and egg tubes and the direction of the vagina. The illustrations have an authenticity so lacking in the nude drawings seen in booklets put out by the medical profession, which invariably show a slim well-rounded woman in her twenties with downcast eyes standing in a demure pose.

Suzann's illustrations of women's internal structures are based on her study of drawings from English, German, French and Italian texts, most of which are not to scale, and which invariably leave out certain structures so that other structures can be seen. Self-helpers translated the material so that Suzann could combine careful reading with our continuous discussions and self-examinations. Still, she has had to infer much, particularly in her drawings of the clitoris, since an extensive study of many anatomy and sex education books revealed no cross section of the clitoris.

To produce the photographs, Sylvia Morales photographed over a hundred women's cervixes, vulvas, clitorises and hair patterns. Each photograph was coded with the woman's name and a brief medical history to identify particular features shown in the photograph. By experimentation with lighting and various types of lenses, Sylvia produced the best cervix photographs ever—containing more information than many photographs in medical texts.

As word of our writing and research spread, we were asked to teach a course called "Women and Their Bodies" in the Women's Studies Department of California State University at Long Beach. The goal of the course is to give women tools to understand their physiology and sexuality and to acquaint them with crucial issues in women's health care. We also became active in the National Women's Studies Association and have shared our course materials, our methods of self-examination and our views on feminist health care at its national conferences.

Full Circle

We first intended to throw together quickly a collection of photographs, a few drawings and a sampling of our literature. We called this our "picture book." Five years, two publishers and numerous editors later, our picture book had grown into a virtual encyclopedia on women's health—far too large to be sold at the original modest price. Therefore, we welcomed an offer by Simon and Schuster, who almost ten years ago published the best-selling women's health guide, *Our Bodies, Ourselves,* to produce a book similar to the one we had initially envisioned, featuring Suzann's illustrations and Sylvia's photography. Although this book has lost some material through the process of ruthless selection, we think it has gained enormously in the bold clarity of certain key concepts.

While we have plodded along, writing, discussing, arguing and rewriting, we have seen books on women's health proliferate, but we sincerely believe that you will see that this is the first book since the publication of *Our Bodies, Ourselves* truly to break new ground.

All of the women in all of the health centers who have worked and sacrificed over the years to create this body of knowledge sincerely hope that this new view of a woman's body will change your life in the ways it has changed our lives and the lives of so many women.

2 • Self-Examination

A light, a mirror and a plastic vaginal speculum are the basic tools of self-examination. (A speculum is a device used to look into body cavities and canals. In ancient times, it also meant mirror or body of knowledge.) By inserting the speculum into your vagina and shining a light into the mirror, you can see your cervix, the neck of your uterus. You can also see the os (or opening) in your cervix, where the menstrual blood and other secretions come out; vaginal secretions, if there are any; and the vaginal walls. If you do self-examination throughout your cycle, you might well observe changes in the color of your cervix, which can, for some women, be very dramatic. You might note a difference in texture; for instance, your cervix might be puffy just before your menstrual period. Or you might be able to see any irritations that might be present.

Over the last ten years small groups of women have spread the concept of self-examination throughout the United States and to other parts of the world. They have focused on sharing experiences and information and on exploring normal, healthy differences and common health concerns about menstruation, vaginal conditions, birth control, hormones and menopause, the special concerns of lesbian health and a variety of other topics.

Most medical practitioners focus on disease and emphasize drugs and surgery which all too often have undesirable, even severe, physical effects. They have been uninterested, for the most part, in the extensive benefits of exercise and nutrition, or in sharing cheap, effective self-help remedies with women. For example, many doctors have ignored the most widely known self-help remedy for a yeast condition—yogurt—in favor of strong vaginal creams, which they admit won't necessarily do more than suppress the symptoms. Many doctors are also oriented toward high profit, so that people's ability to pay directly influences the quality of health care they receive.

The self-help approach, which differs from the popular self-care movement that places the responsibility for health maintenance solely on the individual, directly challenges physicians' control of routine health care and healing, especially women's reproductive health.

Self-help has also developed the role of the patient advocate, a health worker or friend who supports and promotes the rights and decisions of someone who is undergoing medical treatment. Another important aspect of this approach is the insistence on informed consent; that is, that people have full information about their condition, as well as all of the possible adverse effects of any treatment that is planned, so that they can decide what risks they are willing to take.

Every woman's body is different, but whatever your age, ethnic background, economic situation or sexual orientation, you can learn from self-examination. Women will soon be able to buy a plastic vaginal speculum as easily as a toothbrush, in any drugstore or supermarket (maybe even in department stores), and, through its use, begin to acquire knowledge about their bodies and health that has, for years, been solely in the possession of physicians.

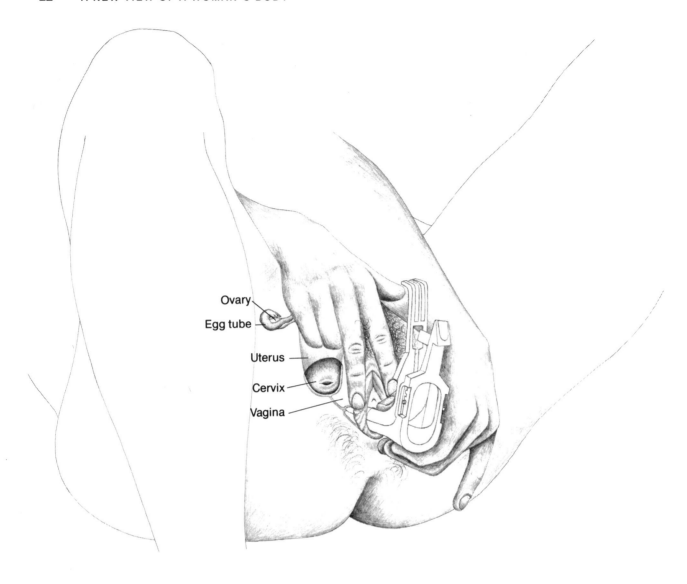

Ovary

Egg tube

Uterus

Cervix

Vagina

2-1   A woman inserting a speculum

Vaginal and Cervical
Self-Examination

Vaginal and cervical self-examination is one of the most useful health tools a woman can have. It enables us to see a vital part of our anatomy which is hidden from plain view—the vagina and cervix, which is the neck of the womb. By using a speculum, you can observe changes in your cervix, secretions, the menstrual cycle and indications of fertility; you can identify and treat common vaginal conditions such as yeast, trichomonas or bacterial infections (which often cause itching or discharge); and you can learn what your cervix looks like day by day, rather than depending on a physician to look once a year to pronounce what is normal for you.

2-1 To insert a plastic speculum, spread the inner lips of the clitoris with two fingers of one hand, hold the bills of the speculum tightly together with the

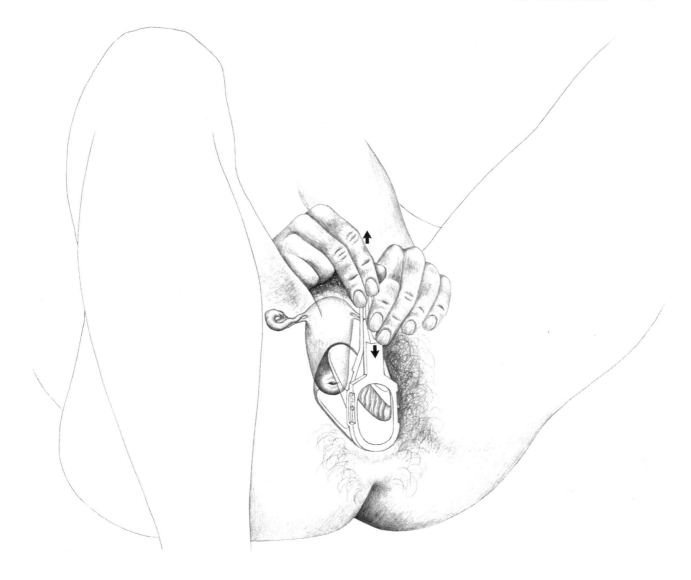

2–2   A woman opening a speculum

thumb and index finger of the other and guide it into the vaginal canal. You can use a water-soluble jelly or just plain water to make insertion smoother. This woman is inserting her speculum with the handles upright, but some women prefer to insert it sideways initially. Inserting the speculum with the handles down is strictly for the doctor's convenience, and it requires that a woman put her feet into stirrups at the end of an exam table.

Speculums can be bought in bulk from a surgical supply company, at some women's bookstores or from women's health projects. (See Appendix.)

2–2 When the handles of the speculum are pinched together, they force the bills open, stretching the vaginal walls and revealing the cervix. With the handles held tightly together, the short handle slides down and the long handle slides up. When there is a sharp click, the speculum is locked into place.

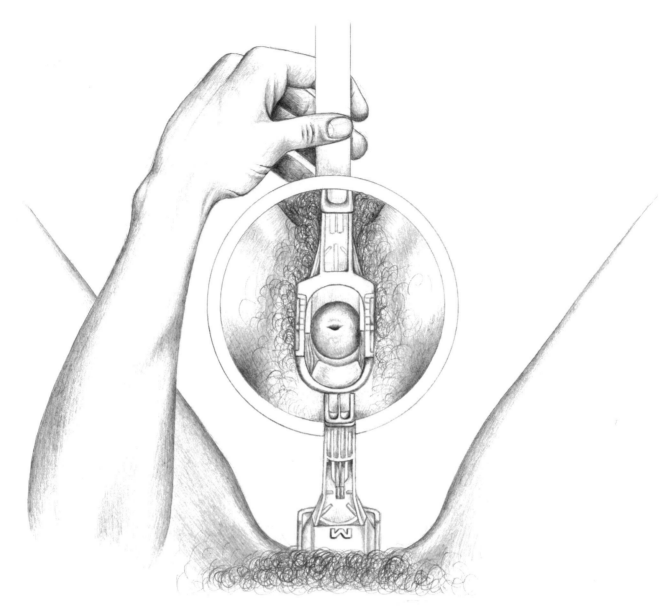

2–3 A view of the cervix in a mirror

2–3 With the speculum locked, both hands are free to hold a mirror and a flashlight or gooseneck lamp. If a flashlight is used, the beam shines *into the mirror* and it will, in turn, be reflected into the vagina, illuminating the vaginal walls and the cervix.

The cervix won't always pop instantly into view. Sometimes you have to try several times. If it stubbornly refuses to appear, you can move around or jump up and down a few times. Sometimes it is also helpful to move to a firmer surface, like the floor or a tabletop. When the cervix is visible, you can see a rounded or flattened knob, between the size of a quarter and a 50-cent piece, like a fat donut with a hole or slit in it. The hole, called the cervical os, is where the menstrual blood, other uterine secretions and babies come out.

Your cervix might be pink and smooth, or it might have a few reddish blemishes. It can also be uneven, rough or splotchy. In any case, the only time to worry is when abnormal cells are found in a Pap smear. The variation in the appearances of women's cervixes is illustrated in the color section of this book.

2–4 Plastic vaginal speculums come in narrow, medium and long. The narrow is as long as the medium, but not as wide. The long is the same width as the medium, but longer.

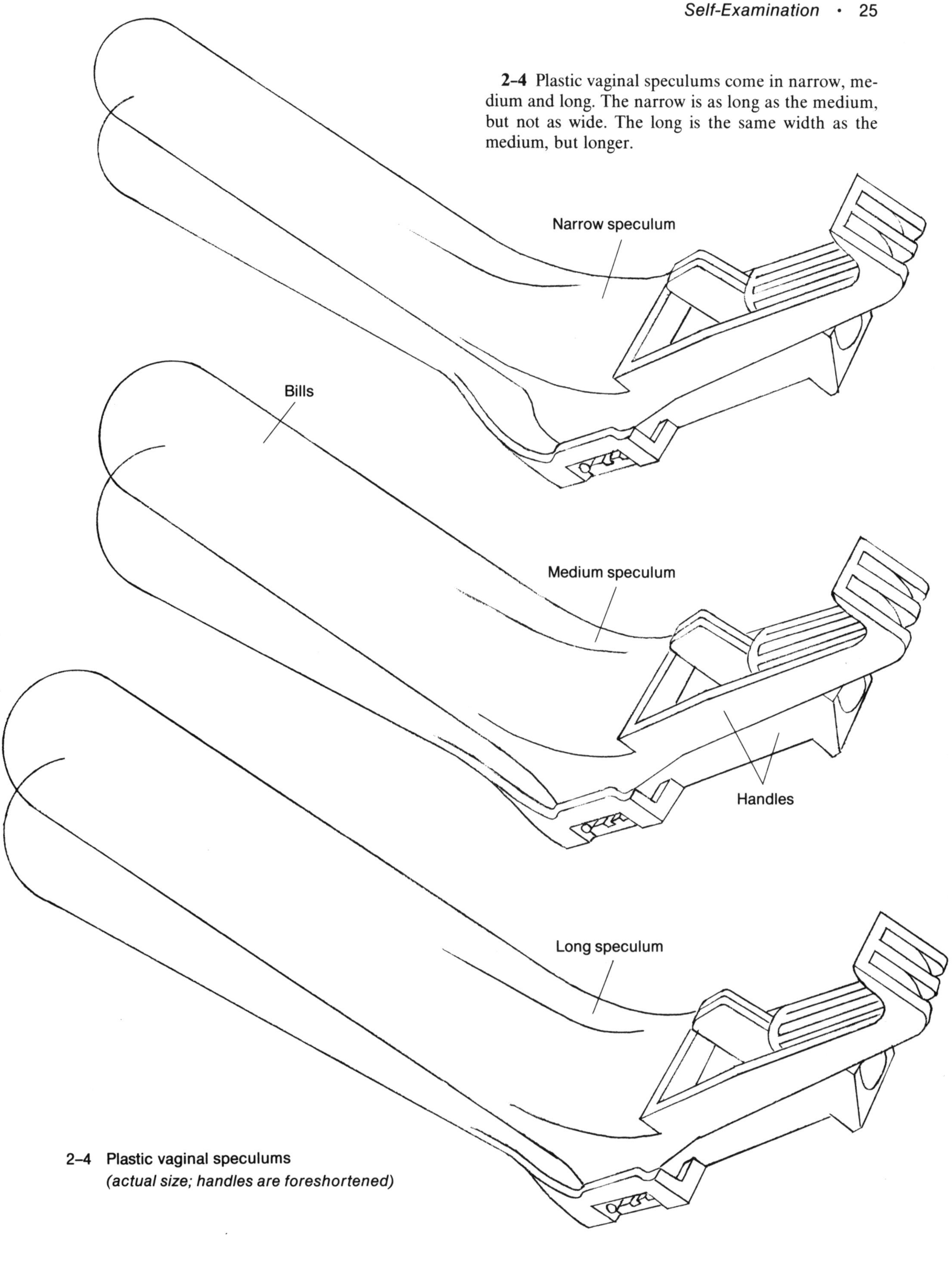

Narrow speculum

Bills

Medium speculum

Handles

Long speculum

2–4 Plastic vaginal speculums
(actual size; handles are foreshortened)

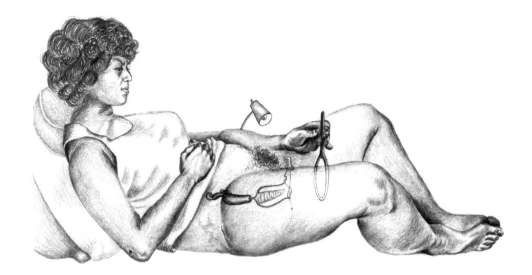

2–5 A woman doing self-examination with a medium
       speculum (incorrect size)

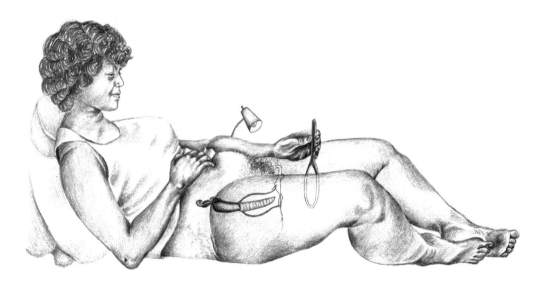

2–6 A woman doing self-examination with a long
       speculum (correct size)

2-5 This woman is using a medium speculum, which is not long enough to expose her cervix. We've used a see-through technique to let you see through this woman's thigh to the speculum's position in her body.

2-6 Here, the same woman is doing self-examination in a slightly different position, using a long speculum. Now she can see her cervix. Self-helpers have observed that the size of a woman's vagina has no relation to her height or weight, or whether or not she has had children.

2-7, 2-8 Breast self-examination is one of the most widely used and vitally important health-care techniques available to women. Every woman is more familiar with the variations and nuances of her body than any doctor can be at an annual examination. Many doctors, in fact, do not check the breasts as part of routine examinations. This is one reason, no doubt, that 90 percent of all breast lumps are found by women themselves. If a lump is discovered, you have several options for diagnosis and treatment. (See the section on breast surgery in Chapter 10.) Although breast self-examination can be done at any time of the month, many women find it easiest to check for suspicious lumps a few days after a period ends. The breasts are least likely to be affected by the hormone cycle then.

Although the steps in a breast self-exam can be done in any order, many women have a routine and follow it closely. The most important thing is to be systematic and thorough. There are two parts to the exam: first, to look for changes on or just under the surface of the skin and second, to feel for lumps deeper under the surface.

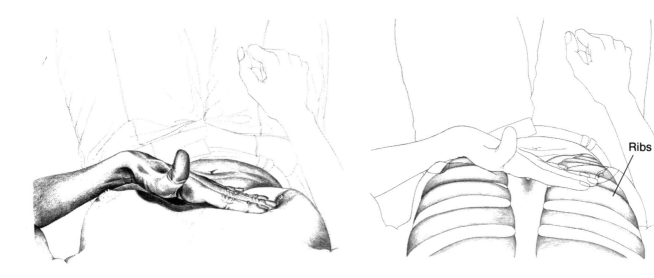

2–7   A woman's-eye view of breast self-examination

2–8   A woman feeling her ribs through her breast

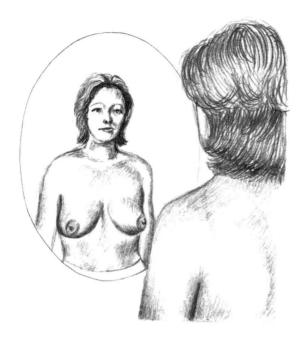

2-9   A woman looking in a mirror

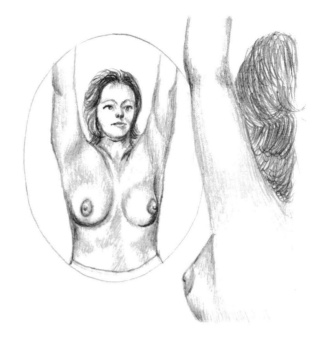

2-10   A woman raising her arms while looking in a mirror

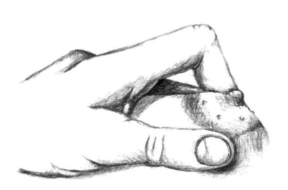

2-11   Squeezing the nipple

2-9 Although the easiest place to do the visual part of the exam is in front of a mirror, it can be done without one. You are checking each breast for rough or raised patches of skin, a change in direction of a nipple, changes in moles or changes in the size or shape of either breast.

2-10 Then raise your arms and check for places where the skin pulls or seems tight. It is quite normal for one breast to be larger than the other or for the nipples to face in different directions. Nipples that sink in instead of pointing out (doctors call them "inverted nipples") are not uncommon, nor are they abnormal (unless they were not previously inverted).

2-11 Sometimes, squeezing the nipples may cause a tiny bit of fluid to appear. Occasionally, a few drops of clear or whitish liquid may come out. If the liquid is bloody, green or forms a crust, you may have an infection that needs treatment. Models in fashion magazines don't have hair around their nipples, but many women do—a little or quite a bit.

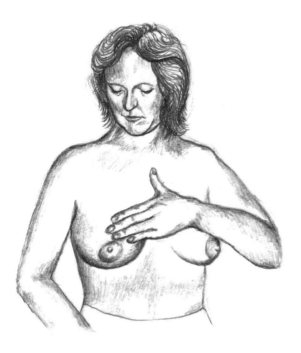

2–12 A woman feeling the upper part of her breast

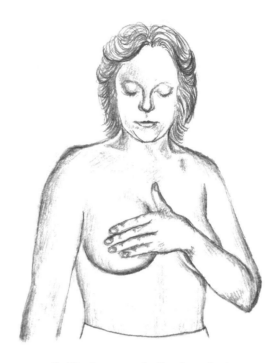

2–13 A woman feeling her nipple

2-12 Next, check one side and then the other, feeling the entire area of the breast with the flat part of the index and middle fingers, being careful not to miss any part.

2-13 Some women feel every part of the breast in a circular motion until they have covered all of it. Others feel the breast in pie-shaped wedges, working from the nipple out, until they've checked the whole breast.

2-14 The breast tissue extends from the side of the rib cage through the entire armpit area to the chest muscles above the breast. Check for enlarged lymph nodes in the armpit, which can be associated with a cancerous growth in the breast. (These nodes can also become swollen and tender from viruses or other infections, but this is not necessarily serious.) Underneath the breast, there is a ridge of tissue which sometimes feels like a lump or growth. It is, in fact, only a band of muscles attached to the chest walls to help support the breast.

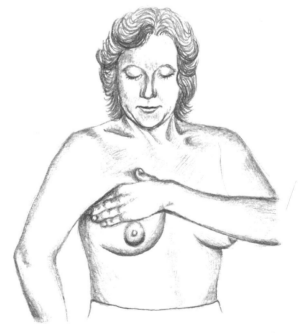

2–14 A woman feeling her armpit

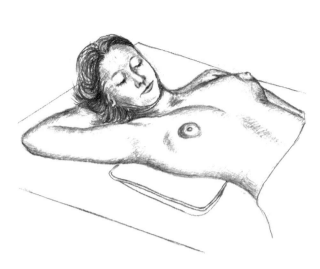

2–15 A woman lying down with a pillow under her shoulder

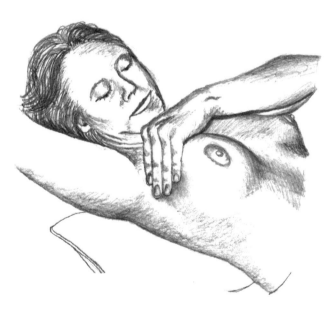

2–16 A woman feeling the upper part of her breast while lying down

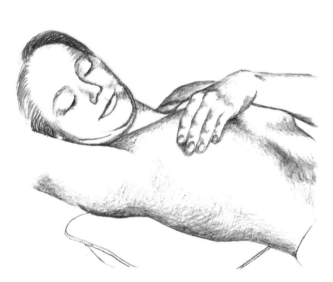

2–17 A woman feeling her nipple while lying down

2–18 A woman feeling her armpit while lying down

2-15 If you have large breasts, you can more easily feel for lumps or changes if you lie on a bed or other flat surface and place a folded towel or small pillow under your shoulder.

2-16 With your hand tucked behind your head, the breast spreads out so that you can more accurately feel the various parts. Thin women can feel their ribs and sometimes mistake a bone for a suspicious lump.

2-17 In self-help groups, women often remark that the interior of the breast feels strange. The breasts have milk glands and ducts, muscles, fat deposits and perhaps cysts, which are almost always harmless. Women are often told that they have "cystic breasts" or notice themselves that they have large, lumpy fat deposits. By doing regular breast self-exam, a woman can know what is normal for herself.

2-18 It isn't easy to distinguish between a lump that might be cancerous and one that is harmless. Be

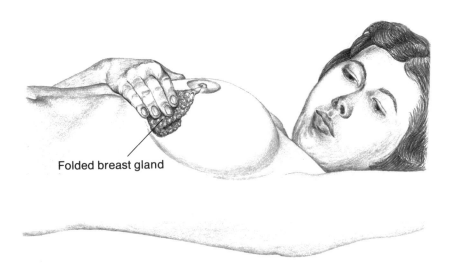

2–19 A woman lying on her back feeling a folded breast gland

suspicious of a lump that is a hard mass that doesn't move, or one that seems to grow into surrounding tissue or is attached to the chest wall. Be less concerned about a self-contained, fluid-filled mass, like a cyst, which might feel like a peeled grape, or of fatty, fibrous tumors which can hurt when you squeeze them. When a lump is first detected, it might be helpful to consult a health worker or a doctor who can evaluate it based on their experience in doing many breast exams.

2–19 Here, a woman is feeling the ridge at the bottom of her breast where her milk glands have folded over. Women who have large breasts are most likely to find this type of growth, which can be mistaken for a lump.

2–20 Some women have stretch marks, which can be caused by normal breast growth or growth caused by the Pill, gain and loss of weight, or pregnancy and nursing. Some women have found that applying cream or vitamin E oil, cocoa butter or other skin moisturizers helps to reduce the severity of the marks, but there is no magic way to make them disappear. There doesn't seem to be any simple explanation of why some people get very distinct, sometimes deeply colored, stretch marks and some don't. For some women, the stretch marks of pregnancy or weight loss will disappear entirely and, for others, they only fade and become less noticeable.

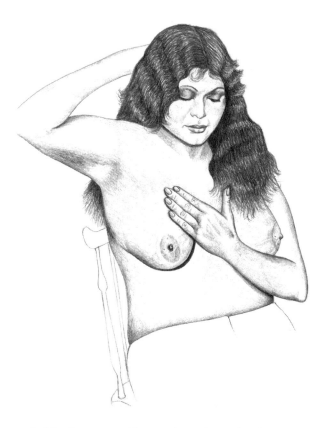

2–20 A woman with stretch marks on her breasts

3. The Clitoris: A Feminist Perspective

Self-Examination of a Woman's Sexual Organ—The Clitoris

Of all aspects of women's health, sexuality has been the most neglected. Other than the work of William H. Masters and Virginia Johnson, the little investigation that has been undertaken has been done mainly by men whose information comes from medical textbooks, also written by men, from medical practice which is centered on illness and disease, and from the authors' own limited personal experience. In standard medical texts you can find a few paragraphs devoted to women's genitals, while many pages are devoted to the penis. Most medical illustrators are men—which perhaps explains why there have been intricate cross sections of the penis since Leonardo da Vinci's time, while comparable drawings of the female organs often have areas of *empty space!* Distortions can be seen in almost any drawing. For example, the vagina is almost always shown as a gaping hole or an open tunnel, which it is not.

There are also deeply entrenched myths that have been perpetuated by the medical profession, sex educators and sex therapists. The myth of the vaginal orgasm. The idea that there is some "correct" way for women to achieve orgasm. The idea that the clitoris consists of only three parts: the glans, hood and shaft. The notion that women's sexual response is somehow totally dependent upon stimulation by a penis. Even the current women's health guides contain abbreviated descriptions of the clitoris—a fact which unwittingly perpetuates a male bias.

As feminists, we wanted to remedy the neglect of women's sexuality and the misdirection of the interests of physicians and sex researchers. As part of a study with this purpose, we took off our pants and compared ourselves with illustrations in the most respected anatomy texts, both American and European. We found that we did have all of the parts of the clitoris shown, and *more.* Besides, not one of these drawings hinted at the wide variation in texture, size and color that we observed. We also observed the changes that occur during the sexual-response cycle when some of the study participants masturbated to orgasm. Then we compared our life experiences to the textbook version. Using self-examination, personal observation and meticulous analysis, we arrived at *a new view of the clitoris.*

We were pleased to learn that the clitoris has many distinct parts in addition to its visible structures, such as bodies of erectile tissue, muscle, nerves and blood vessels. The exterior of the clitoris, which is bounded by the hairy outer lips of the vulva, is easy to distinguish because its intricate, fleshly structures are hairless. These structures swell slightly when sexually stimulated. Beneath them are several spongy masses which fill with blood and swell greatly as sexual tension heightens, and layers of muscles which contract in unison at orgasm, forcing the accumulated blood back into the body. This entire complex organ is richly supplied with blood vessels and nerve endings.

Before we made painstaking comparisons of our sexual anatomy to the drawings we found in medical texts and discussed them at length, our knowledge of our sexual response was quite hazy. We knew that the feminist movement, backed by Masters and Johnson's research, had debunked Freud and stated that the clitoris (defined merely as a tiny, ball-like bump, shaft and hood just outside the vagina) was the site of female pleasure. But, beyond that, we didn't really know why or how some women achieve orgasm, why some women don't, or precisely what an orgasm is.

Since we had no access to dissection rooms, we were forced to rely on Masters and Johnson's research, anatomy texts, the drawings of Robert Dickinson (an artist-physician who interviewed and sketched thousands of his patients in the 1920s and 1930s), and the observation of our own bodies.

We felt that Masters and Johnson failed to describe the clitoris fully and instead designated most clitoral structures as being somehow an extension of the vagina called the "orgasmic platform" located in the outer third of the vagina. Even though it was an advance for them to identify the glans as the focal point of sexual pleasure, they still essentially ignored the rest of the clitoris. Mary Jane Sherfey, whose book, *The Nature and Evolution of Female Sexuality,* is based largely on Masters and Johnson, was the first to consider the clitoris as being more extensive than the glans and shaft.

The research for the illustrations in this chapter was done by Carol Downer, Suzann Gage, Sherry Schiffer, Lorraine Rothman, Francie Hornstein, Lynn Heidelberg and Kathleen Hodge in Los Angeles. Additional research was done by Lynn Walker, Chris Cleary and Nancy Walker in Orange County, California.

3–1 The inner lips are parallel folds of skin inside the hair-covered outer lips. By spreading them apart

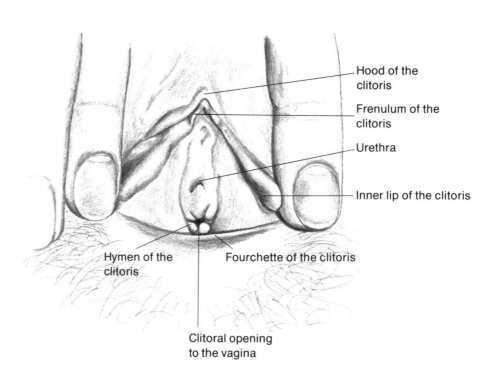

Hood of the clitoris

Frenulum of the clitoris

Urethra

Inner lip of the clitoris

Hymen of the clitoris

Fourchette of the clitoris

Clitoral opening to the vagina

3–1 An outer view of the clitoris

with your fingers, you can see the exterior parts of your clitoris. The hood is formed by the joining of the inner lips, like a tent, over the glans and shaft. One, perhaps two, small folds of skin which form an inverted "V" where the inner lips meet is called the frenulum. Its appearance can vary greatly from woman to woman. Below is the opening to the urethra, a short tube which leads to the bladder. This opening is often difficult to locate because it is extremely small and can be hidden in the folds of tissue. It can be very close to the vaginal opening. Below that is the clitoral opening to the vagina. In this drawing done from life, it is an elastic opening formed by closely folded tissue. About an inch within the opening is the hymen, either a ring of toothy projections or, in young girls and some adult women, a membrane greatly or almost completely stretched across the entrance to the vagina.

The inner lips are thinner than the dusky-colored outer lips, feel smooth inside and have veins which can be seen through the skin. The shading can range from bright red or pink on the inside to deep brown or black on the outer part and their texture can be crinkly or more like folds of skin.

The lips vary in size from woman to woman. They can sometimes be larger than the outer lips and, in fact, one side can be larger than the other. The membrane at the bottom of the lips, called the fourchette, is like a thin curtain stretched from one side to the other. Its appearance can vary a great deal, and some women who have had episiotomies during childbirth may not have one at all.

3-2 Pulling back the hood, which is formed by the meeting of the inner lips, reveals the glans of the clitoris, a smooth, round bump, somewhat hard to find but highly sensitive to the touch. This action also stretches out the skin directly above and attached to the hood, the front commissure. Many women find that direct pressure on this spot with the flat of the fingers in a round or back-and-forth motion is the most effective way to stimulate the shaft of the clitoris.

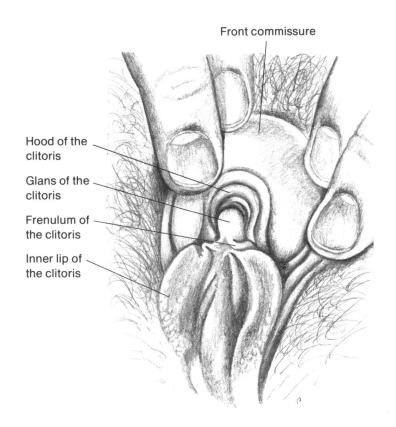

Front commissure

Hood of the clitoris

Glans of the clitoris

Frenulum of the clitoris

Inner lip of the clitoris

3-2　The glans of the clitoris

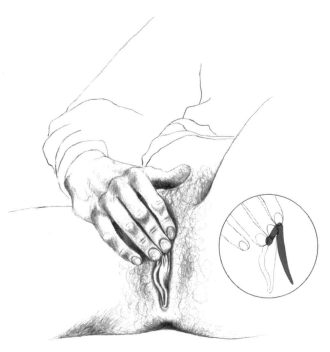

3-3 Sitting on the floor or on any other firm surface, you can locate the glans and shaft of the clitoris by feeling. Here, this woman places her fourth finger at the point where the inner lips meet and gently presses down. As the inset shows, she can feel the glans with her fourth finger and her middle and index fingers rest on the shaft.

3-3 A woman doing self-examination of the clitoris by rolling the shaft

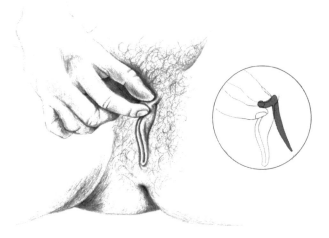

3-4 It is also possible to feel the glans and shaft of the clitoris by placing the index finger where the inner lips meet and the thumb above the hood of the clitoris, and squeezing. The shaft, which feels like a round rubber cord, usually moves easily when you press it.

3-4 A woman doing self-examination of the clitoris by squeezing the glans

3-5 If you look in a mirror, you can see your vulva, a fatty layer of skin covered by pubic hair. This black woman's vulva surrounds and protects the clitoris. In addition to the pubic mound, the vulva includes the outer lips and the anus, which are darker in color than the clitoris itself or the skin surrounding it. The visible parts of the clitoris in this illustration are the hood; the frenulum, where the skin of the inner lips meets at the glans; the clitoral opening to the vagina; the hymen; the fourchette; the perineum; and the urethra.

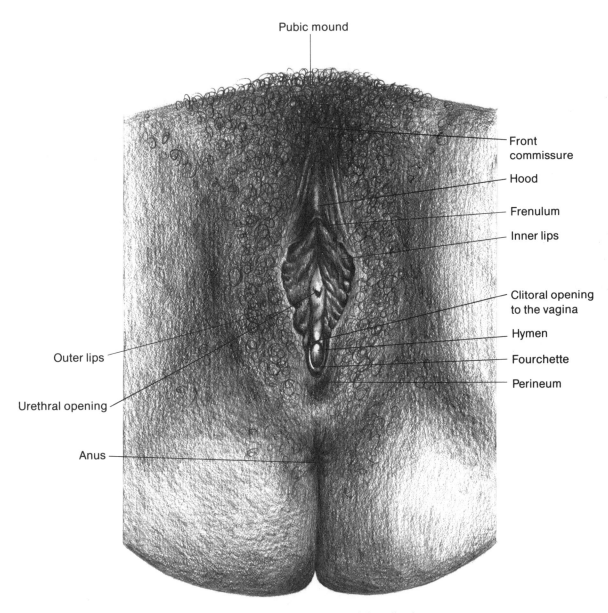

Pubic mound

Front commissure

Hood

Frenulum

Inner lips

Clitoral opening to the vagina

Hymen

Fourchette

Perineum

Outer lips

Urethral opening

Anus

3–5 The outer anatomy of the clitoris

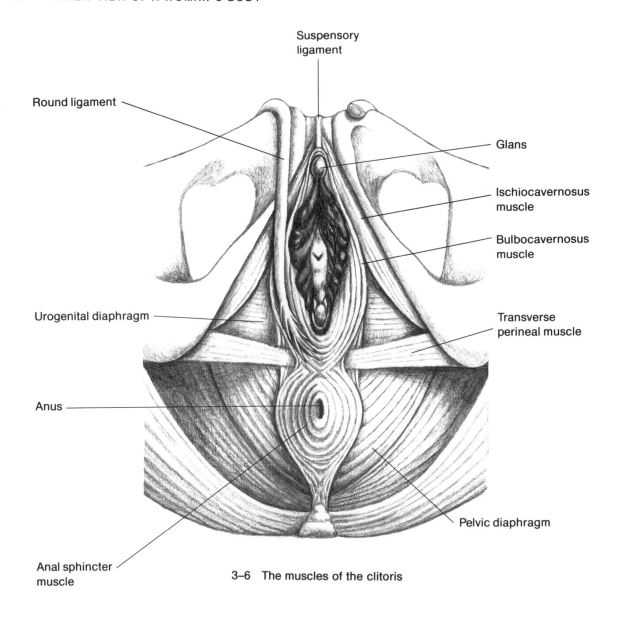

Suspensory ligament

Round ligament

Glans

Ischiocavernosus muscle

Bulbocavernosus muscle

Urogenital diaphragm

Transverse perineal muscle

Anus

Anal sphincter muscle

Pelvic diaphragm

3–6   The muscles of the clitoris

3–6 Beneath the pubic mound the pelvic bones flare out forming a triangular space, called the pelvic outlet, which is generally wider than in men. During birth the baby passes through this outlet.

Two pairs of long slender muscles frame the pelvic outlet. One pair (the ischiocavernosus) runs alongside the pelvic bones, forming the two sides of the triangle, with the glans of the clitoris at its apex. The other pair (the transverse perineal muscles) extends laterally from the perineum and connects these muscles, forming the base of the triangle. A third pair of muscles (the bulbocavernosus) also extends from the glans of the clitoris within the triangle downward under the outer lips, connecting at the perineum. You can locate these muscles by squeezing as if you wanted to stop the flow of urine or a bowel movement.

During orgasm, these muscles, which lie just beneath the top layer of skin and fat, all contract in unison, compressing the soft, engorged tissues of the clitoris between them. At the same time, they compress the more interior tissues between themselves and the underlying broad layers of muscles.

A small ligament divides the cartilage where the pubic bones meet. It is attached to the clitoral shaft and draws it and the glans up during sexual arousal. The round ligament of the uterus (or womb) runs along each side of the lips of the clitoris.

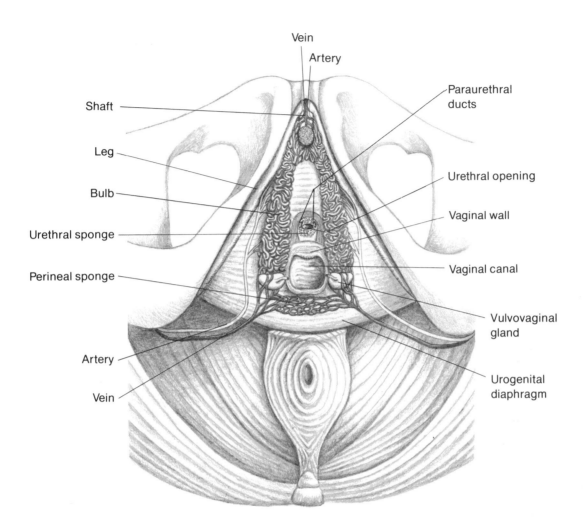

3-7 The erectile tissue of the clitoris

3-7 Through self-examination, you can locate many of the structures which lie beneath the surface of the skin.

Under the top layer of muscles lies a layer of erectile tissue and blood vessels. In the clitoris, there are two types of erectile tissue: one is more firm and the other is more elastic. When filled with blood during sexual excitement, they both become firmer and support erection. The blood that fills these intricate, tightly packed compartments of tiny arteries and veins comes from larger arteries.

The shaft and legs of the clitoris are long, thin bands of the firm tissue which flare outward from the shaft along the pubic bones. The bulb of the clitoris, which is underneath the outer lips and top layer of muscle, is made up of the more elastic tissue. Another spongy body, extends inward along the ceiling of the vagina. This pad of soft tissue can be easily located by inserting your finger into the vagina and pressing forward toward the pubic bone; it surrounds the urethra, undoubtedly protecting it from direct pressure during sexual activity. This structure was not named in textbooks so we called it the "urethral sponge."

There are two sets of glands within the clitoris which have ducts that open to the outside. One set are minute and their specific function, if any, is unknown. The other, the vulvovaginal glands, do secrete a few drops of fluid during sexual arousal. Usually, a woman becomes aware of these latter glands only if they become infected and enlarged.

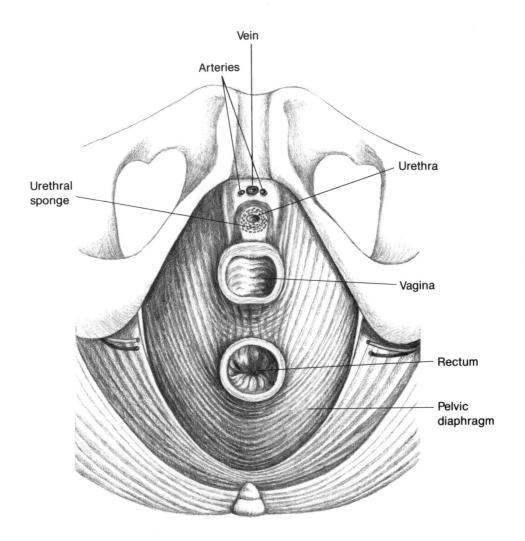

3–8 The pelvic muscles (without the clitoris)

In doing self-examination to explore the clitoris, we noticed an area between the vagina and the anus that "gives" when you press on it. This we discovered to be erectile tissue which forms the lower part of the clitoris to a depth of an inch or so. Lacking any medical labels, we have called this the "perineal sponge."

3–8 Attached to either side of the flared pelvic bones and wrapped around both the rectum and vagina is the pelvic diaphragm, a voluntary muscle. All the structures of the clitoris rest on this large muscle which tightens the rectum and vagina when contracted. Dr. Arnold Kegal of Los Angeles has drawn attention to this muscle, the pubococcygeal, by advocating that it be strengthened to increase sexual pleasure. He recommends that, several times a day, you repeatedly contract this muscle as if to stop the flow of urine or bowel movement. Childbirth educators also suggest this and similar exercises to make this muscle and the other muscles of the clitoris stronger and more elastic.

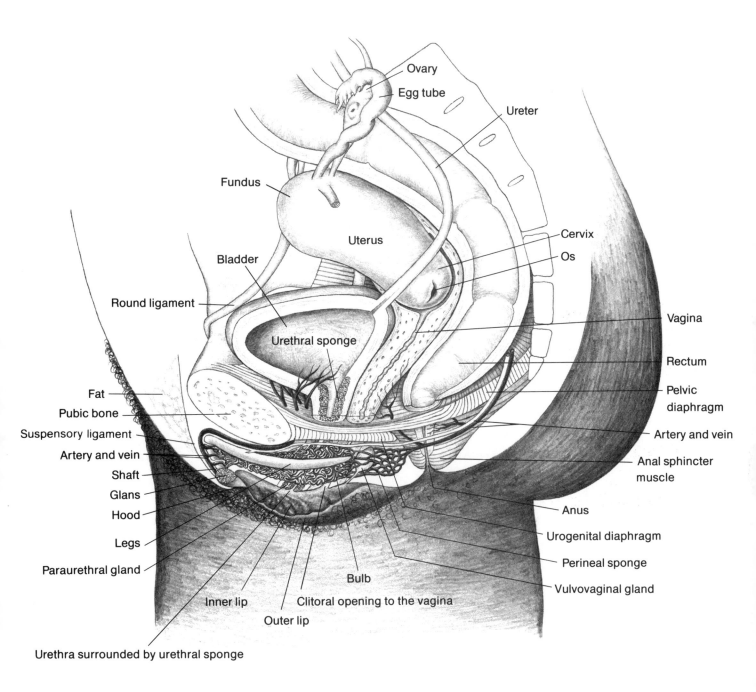

Ovary
Egg tube
Ureter
Fundus
Cervix
Uterus
Bladder
Os
Round ligament
Vagina
Urethral sponge
Rectum
Fat
Pelvic diaphragm
Pubic bone
Suspensory ligament
Artery and vein
Artery and vein
Shaft
Anal sphincter muscle
Glans
Hood
Anus
Legs
Urogenital diaphragm
Paraurethral gland
Perineal sponge
Bulb
Vulvovaginal gland
Inner lip
Clitoral opening to the vagina
Outer lip
Urethra surrounded by urethral sponge

3–9   A cross section of the clitoris

3-9 In all of the anatomy and sex education books we studied, there were several cross sections of the penis, but *no cross section of the clitoris.* This cross section shows very clearly the organs and other muscles involved in sexual response. The clitoris is in a nonerect, nonexcited state.

Not shown are the clitoral muscles which are very much involved in orgasm.

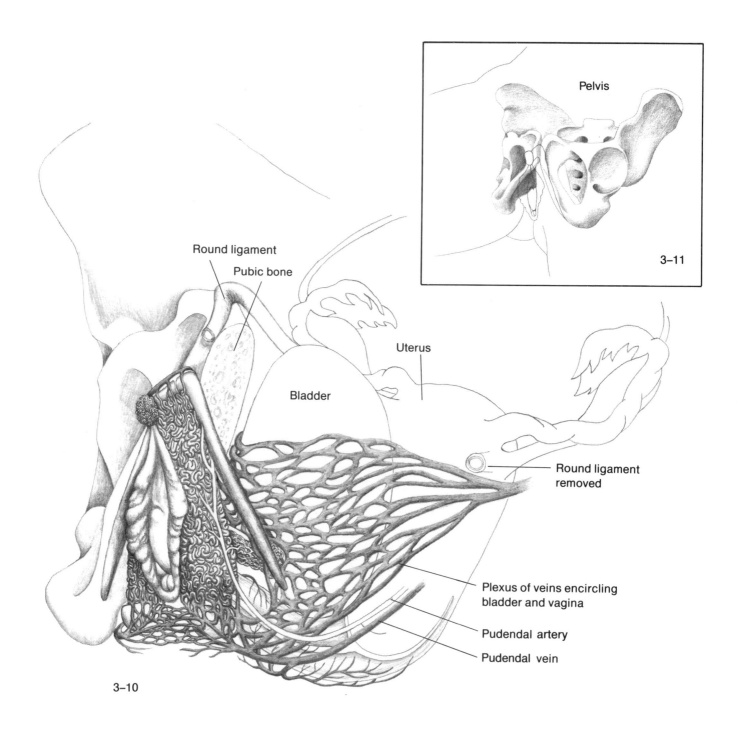

Pelvis

3–11

Round ligament

Pubic bone

Uterus

Bladder

Round ligament
removed

Plexus of veins encircling
bladder and vagina

Pudendal artery

Pudendal vein

3–10

3–10, 3–11 This illustration shows how the clitoris is situated in the pelvis. The inset shows the pelvic bones.

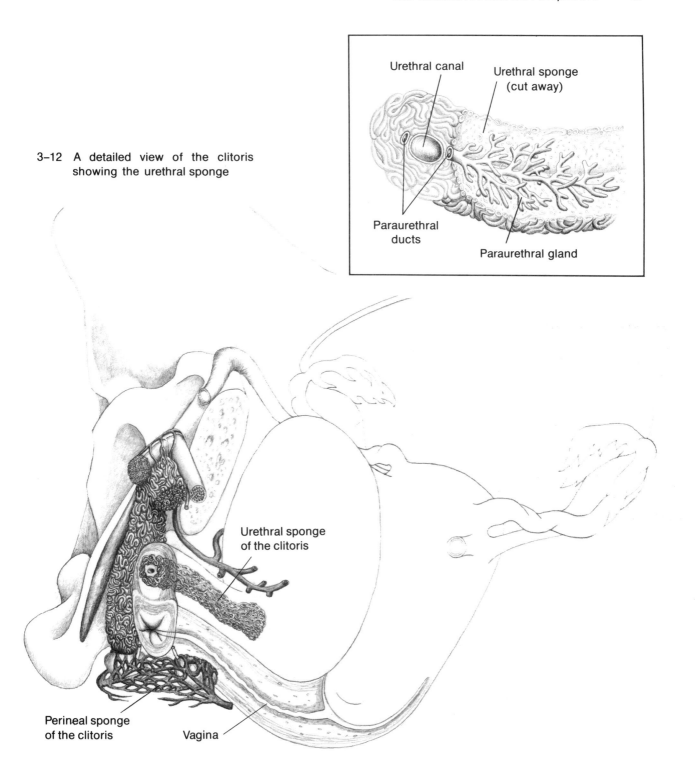

3–12 A detailed view of the clitoris showing the urethral sponge

Urethral canal

Urethral sponge (cut away)

Paraurethral ducts

Paraurethral gland

Urethral sponge of the clitoris

Perineal sponge of the clitoris

Vagina

3-12 This view of the clitoris shows the urethral sponge, which surrounds and protects the urethra. This spongy body fills with blood during sexual excitement and, during coitus, acts as a buffer between the penis and the urethra.

3–13 You can feel the urethral sponge by inserting two fingers into your vagina and pressing back toward the pubic bone. Sometimes, pressing on it can make you feel as if you need to urinate.

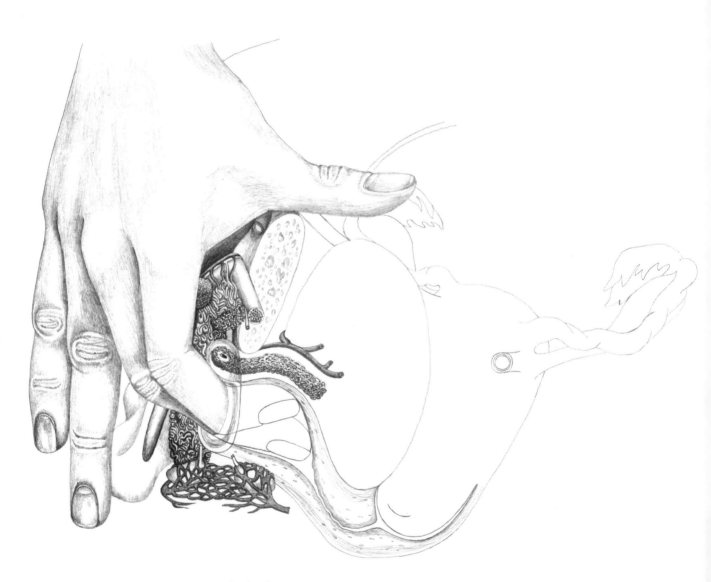

3–13   Self-examination of the urethral sponge

3-14 You can also feel the perineal sponge by inserting your thumb into your vagina and pressing down toward the anus. The tissue compresses, then springs back when the pressure is released. If you try this, you might feel pleasurable sensations in other parts of the clitoris.

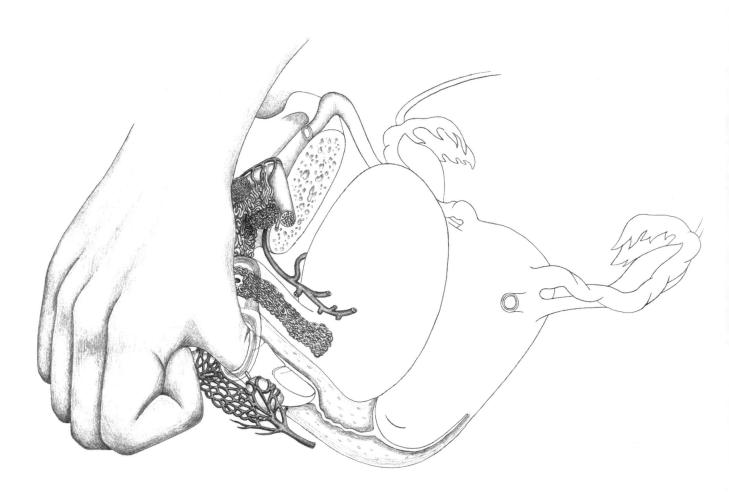

3-14 Self-examination of the perineal sponge

3-15 The nerves which lie in the area of the clitoris are highly concentrated and transmit sensory messages during sexual excitement. The glans has a particularly high concentration of nerves.

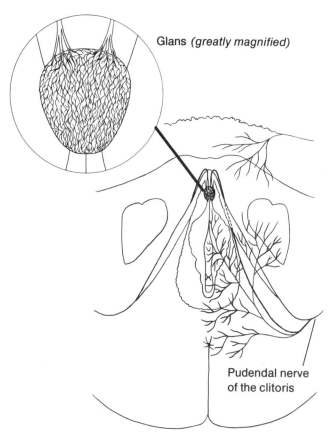

Glans (greatly magnified)

Pudendal nerve of the clitoris

3-15   The nerves of the clitoris

Sexual Response

From the time we are small children, we are discouraged from being familiar with our genitals. We grow up ashamed of our bodies and with the clear impression that the ultimate object of sex is to please men or to have babies.

When a group of us used the self-help approach to learn about women's sexuality, we first studied a wide variety of medical texts, sex manuals and popular literature. We discovered that most sex information is written by men. We felt shortchanged because the information was organized around the penis and didn't account for the full range of women's sexual response. For example, one woman found that, despite having enjoyed years of what she had considered to be satisfactory sex with her husband, she would be classified as frigid by many authorities because she does not

achieve orgasm during coitus, but rather in other ways.

Also, we resented the first stage of the sexual response cycle, excitement, being labeled "foreplay," as though this sexual pleasure was not in itself important, but rather a necessary exercise men needed to go through in order to get us to the plateau and orgasm phases. Naturally, those of us who were celibate or lesbians found it difficult to learn about our bodies' responses when they were portrayed only in terms of a response to male stimulation.

As we did self-examination, exploring the different parts of the clitoris and observing the dynamic changes of sexual response, we realized that, when considered separately, the glans, hood and shaft of the clitoris do resemble a miniature penis, and they have been so described in many a book about sex. However, the problem with such a comparison is that both the male and the female sexual organs consist of a lot more than these parts. The parts of the penis involved in orgasm, such as the powerful muscles that shoot out the semen, are rooted far back in the man's body. (Men whose glans and shaft have been removed surgically can still have orgasms, as do women who have had their glans, hood and shaft removed!) Although they are distinctively different in size and arrangement, the parts of the clitoris are still much the same as the parts of the penis.

In our study, we observed that Masters and Johnson's extremely important discovery—that the male and female sexual responses are similar instead of complementary—applies to the structure and the function of the sex organs as well as to the generalized body responses and changes, such as increased heart rate, rise in blood pressure and respiration, nervous excitement, vasocongestion and muscle tension.

One of the major accomplishments of this group self-study project was to put to rest forever the controversy over clitoral and vaginal orgasms. Now that it is understood that the clitoral structures surround and extend along the vagina, the fact that women report pleasurable feelings deep in the vagina in no way contradicts Masters and Johnson's correct if inadequately examined finding that all orgasms are of clitoral origin. The vagina is involved passively in the orgasm, and the pleasure that women receive from the thrusting of the penis comes from the sensations of the penis rubbing against the erect clitoris.

From Freud to Masters and Johnson, the myth of the vaginal orgasm (which holds that women's orgasms result from vaginal sensations and are, therefore, according to their thinking, dependent upon stimulation from a penis) has been the favorite theory. From our research, we learned that the vigorous contractions of orgasm come from pelvic and clitoral muscles in response to *clitoral* stimulation. By *clitoris* we mean the whole complex organ, consisting of the glans; shaft and hood; clitoral legs (also called crura); inner lips; hymen; several bodies of erectile tissue, including the clitoral bulbs, urethral sponge and perineal sponge; muscles; nerve endings; and networks of blood vessels.

Behind the controversy over vaginal and clitoral orgasm is the tendency of many men to do no more during the actual sex act than thrust an erect penis back and forth in the vagina until they achieve orgasm, and the refusal of women to be forced to rely solely on penile stimulation. Most women do not find this stimulation enough to achieve full sexual satisfaction, no matter what the variation in position, mainly because the clitoris is frequently not fully erect. Whether through mental stimulation, such as the excitement of a new partner, or direct stimulation, particularly of the clitoris, swollen clitoral tissues are far more sensitive to a penis than the vagina itself. Direct stimulation of the commisure, the spot beside and above the shaft, is a favored method for dependable arousal for many women and can be a pleasurable way of achieving orgasm in itself. Masters and Johnson's main point is that *wherever* the final orgasm occurs, clitoral stimulation is a necessary precondition. Our redefinition of the clitoris does not negate this basic assertion.

During coitus, the penis is in contact with part of the clitoris at all times. Despite this contact, many, many healthy women seldom, if ever, have an orgasm during coitus. Many who do experience an orgasm during coitus find that it is necessary to be in a certain position, specifically that of the woman on top, so that they can control the amount and type of stimulation to the pubic mound and glans. Others have orgasms in a variety of positions. Of course, lesbians or any women who masturbate can and do experience well-defined orgasms without coitus. In fact, women have mentioned in self-help groups that they often have more powerful orgasms when they masturbate than when they have sex with a partner.

This redefinition of the clitoris is no mere semantic quibble. Its significance is apparent when it is realized, for example, that if the perineum is part of our sex organ, an episiotomy is more than a surgical incision. It becomes a mutilation of the clitoris. Also, thinking of the clitoris as a functional unit, which it is, is very different from thinking of it as a collection of structures and areas as described by Masters and Johnson. Once understood and recognized, it is clear that the clitoris is an organ as complex and active as the penis. After self-examination of the clitoris, discussions of our sexual experiences become much more concrete and specific. We finally had a vocabulary and conceptual framework with which to communicate.

Another myth that seems ridiculous from a feminist point of view is that there is some correct or socially acceptable way to have an orgasm. Most sex information, for example, focuses on the penis-in-vagina sex act, and implies that orgasms during coitus are the goal of every heterosexual couple. Masturbation is given cursory attention and sex for lesbians or gay men is given superficial attention, if any.

These deeply embedded myths, plus strong social influences, serve to keep women from asserting themselves as fully sexual beings.

Shere Hite's investigation of women's sexuality, detailed in *The Hite Report* and published in 1976, was the first work that approached the topic of sex from a woman's point of view. Hite reported what women themselves thought and felt about their sexuality, not what male doctors and sociologists assume women think. Hite's work plainly reveals that society proscribes or sharply limits women's sexuality as it has their other roles. Hite found that just as women are often expected to serve men as some sort of "household glue," in a more subtle way they are also "sexual slaves" who are always expected to put themselves second. She cites economic dependence as a powerful force in keeping women sexually subservient.

Another critical factor that keeps women from being sexually free is that heterosexual women of childbearing age are forced to depend upon unreliable, hard-to-use, risky methods of birth control. For some women, the fear of pregnancy is so great that they either avoid sex or are too nervous to enjoy it.

We also found that the kind of information available on the physiology of sex was not very meaningful when we tried to apply it to our everyday lives.

Through advertising and the media, we are overwhelmed by images of young, lithe, exquisitely groomed, financially carefree women who bubble with life, the trend of the moment, and love. These ads imply that beautiful, successful women have more fun and, more than likely, better sex. This leaves out poor women, women of color, lesbians, women with physical deformities or disabilities and older women. In other words, women who don't fit the media stereotype. One ironic contradiction we encountered was that while the media ideal for women is slim and svelte, we are not encouraged to be athletic or to do strenuous exercise, which builds strength, encourages overall health and replaces fat and flab with muscle.

This media image also reinforces the view of women as sex objects. Advertisers have zeroed in on the principle that sex sells, and women's bodies are fair game for marketing anything from tequila to motorcycles. Quite often, the faces are dispensed with entirely, so that women become pure *objects* of sexual interest. They are also expected to be available to satisfy men's needs, and then they are *expected* to have orgasms.

Sex is more than having an orgasm. Sex with another person can be the ultimate expression of intimacy. However, it has been our experience that when a woman can connect her subjective experiences with the physiological bases for them, her sexual enjoy-

ment, and that of her partner, is enhanced.

As a part of our research, we gathered accounts of individual experiences. We were more interested in the actual sexual experiences than in feelings about sexuality. We found that some women experience the entire sexual response cycle from the time they are toddlers. On the other hand, it became clear that many women do not experience orgasm until they are in their twenties or thirties, or even later, or never.

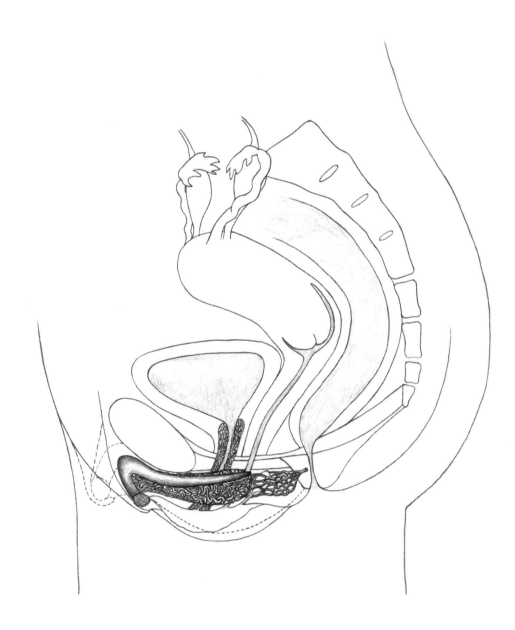

3–16 A side view of the clitoris: Compared to the penis

And we found few women who experience orgasm regularly and dependably during coitus.

This series of drawings of the sexual response cycle provides concrete information about where and how orgasms originate and enables us to understand the functions of our sexual anatomy.

3-16 This is a side view of the clitoris, in a nonerect state. The dotted lines at the left of the drawing show the position of the glans and shaft when they are erect and pulled up beneath the hood. The long dotted line at the bottom shows the position of the clitoral bulb when it is engorged with blood and erect. The spongy area also fills with blood and enlarges greatly during sexual excitement.

3-17 The glans and shaft of the penis are shown here in an unaroused state. The dotted lines show its position when the erectile tissues are filled with blood.

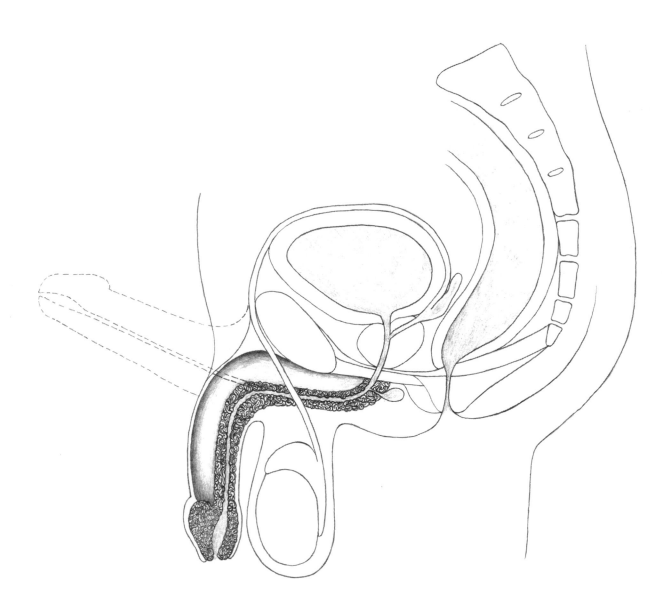

3-17   A side view of the penis: Compared to the clitoris

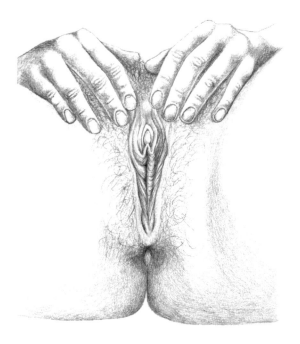

3-18 An outer view of the nonerect clitoris

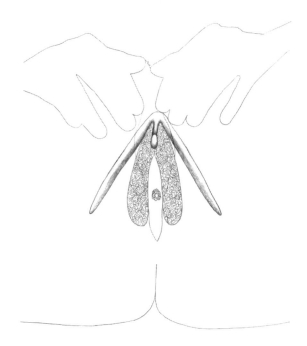

3-19 An inner view of the nonerect clitoris

3-18, 3-19 These illustrations show the clitoris and its underlying tissue in a nonerect state. Here, the glans is nestled among the folds of the hood and is visible because the hood has been pulled back. The woman in this illustration is stimulating the clitoris manually. Her fingers are pressed on either side of the shaft and she is "rocking" her hands, pushing the flesh of the mound back and forth over the pubic bone. Self-help research has shown that many women's clitorises do not look a great deal like standard anatomy-book illustrations.

3-20, 3-21 *Excitement.* The clitoris becomes erect when the underlying spongy bodies fill with blood. This signifies the first, or excitement, stage of sexual response. At the same time, the vagina "sweats," which provides lubrication, the vaginal blood vessels widen and fill with blood and the color of the vaginal walls deepens. At this time there is a noticeable increase in the pulse rate and blood pressure. In most women, the glans is not visible at this point because the shaft has been pulled back by the shortened ligament, causing it to retract from view. She is continuing to apply pressure in rhythmic strokes.

3-22, 3-23 *Plateau.* The bulbs and the urethral sponge become further filled with blood as sexual excitement increases. The valves in the arteries and veins close, trapping the blood in the organ. This is called vasocongestion. The hood enlarges as its supporting ligament shortens and pulls on the shaft, which is now quite hard, and the legs, which have become rigid also. The perineal sponge thickens as it fills with blood, further closing the entrance to the vagina. The uterus, tubes and ovaries swell. The broad ligament, which lies like a blanket over the bladder, swells and tightens, pulling up on the uterus and causing the vagina to enlarge. At this point, her movements have speeded up.

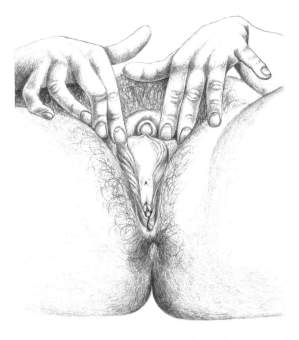

3–20 An outer view of the clitoris during the excitement phase

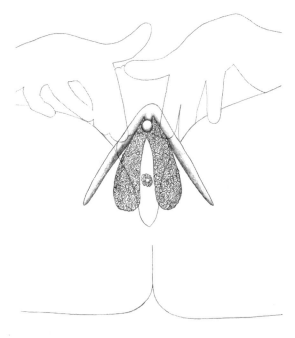

3–21 An inner view of the clitoris during the excitement phase

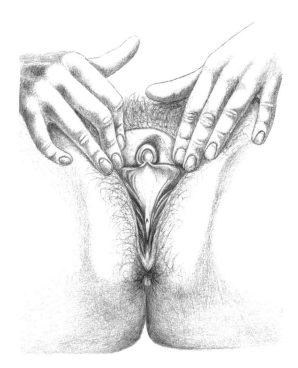

3–22 An outer view of the clitoris during the plateau phase

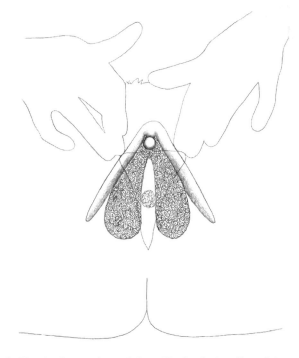

3–23 An inner view of the clitoris during the plateau phase

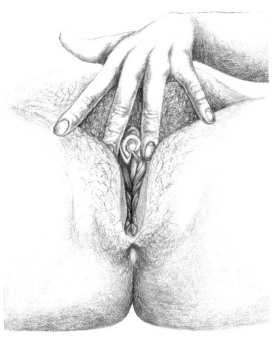

3-24 An outer view of the clitoris during the orgasm phase

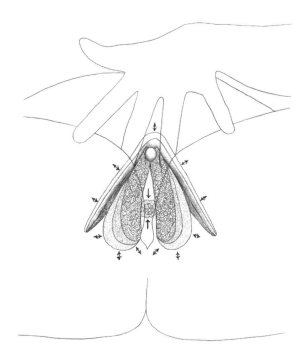

3-25 An inner view of the clitoris during the orgasm phase

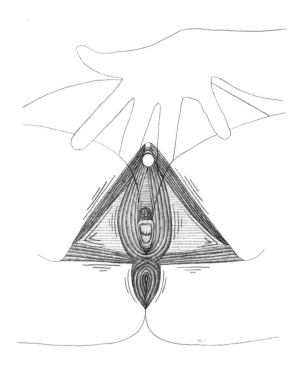

3-26 The clitoral muscles during the orgasm phase

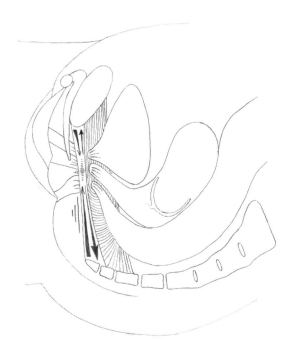

3-27 The pelvic muscles during the orgasm phase

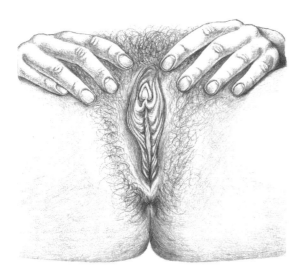

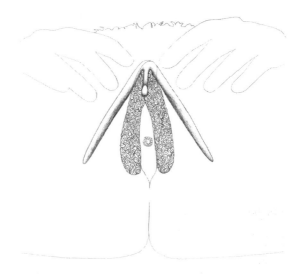

3–28   An outer view of the clitoris during the resolution phase

3–29   An inner view of the clitoris during the resolution phase

3-24, 3-25 *Orgasm.* Powerful, rhythmic muscle contractions begin. The clitoris shortens dramatically and the inner lips tuck in, covering it. These events are accompanied by the loss of voluntary muscle control, faster breathing, tingling sensations and, sometimes, a rash or flush on the breasts and stomach. Some women experience sharp spasms in their hands and feet. Since one of her hands has become tired, she continues and intensifies the pressure with the other until orgasm.

3-26 During sexual arousal, the muscular structure of the clitoris becomes very active. The muscles shown here tighten and, during orgasm, contract involuntarily.

3-27 During orgasm, the sling of muscle tissue suspended between the pubic bone and coccyx stretches taut and contracts involuntarily, constricting the vaginal opening, urethra and rectum.

3-28, 3-29 *Resolution.* The contractions of the clitoris prevent blood from flooding the tissues further. The tissues shrink as the pulse rate lowers, the valves in the arteries and veins open and the inner lips return to their original color. Within seconds, the orgasmic contractions grow faint and fade away. She is relaxed and covered with a fine film of perspiration.

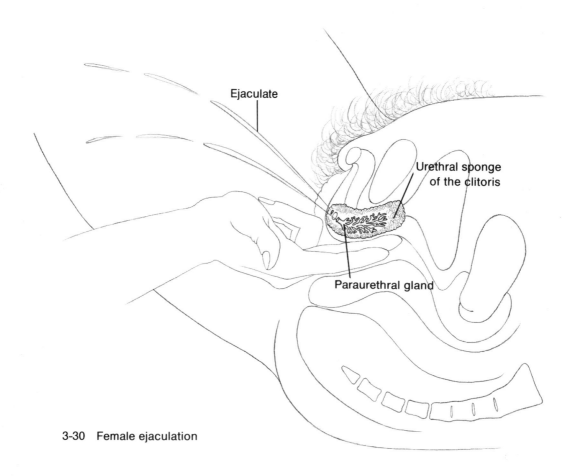

Ejaculate

Urethral sponge of the clitoris

Paraurethral gland

3-30   Female ejaculation

3-30 Some self-helpers have reported that occasionally fluid squirts from their clitorises when they have an orgasm. This fluid shoots out like a stream in bursts. One woman described this phenomenon as "gallons" of fluid, distinct from vaginal sweating. Some women have confused this with urination. One woman noted that the fluid had an odor different from urine. Unlike the involuntary urination that occurs in a small number of women during sex, this fluid is chemically different from urine and appears to be ejaculated from the paraurethral glands located in the urethral sponge of the clitoris. The same structure that becomes the paraurethral glands in the female during fetal development becomes the prostate gland in the male, which later contributes to the male ejaculate. A group of lesbians, having had this experience, related their observations to sex researchers Beverly Whipple, R.N., and John Perry, Ph.D. In reviewing the literature, Whipple and Perry found that a researcher named Grafenberg had reported similar findings in the early 1950s. He acknowledged the presence of highly sensitive and spongy tissue surrounding the urethra and noted that direct stimulation of this tissue could result in a release of fluid during orgasm which did not appear to be urine. Based on this research and their own clinical observations, Whipple and Perry concluded that these women were experiencing female ejaculation and coined the phrase "Grafenberg spot" to identify what they believed to be the site of stimulation and ejaculation in the vagina. The rediscovery of clitoral tissue around the urethra and paraurethral glands reveals that stimulation of the clitoris is integral to this response. In addition to ejaculation, some self-helpers have said that stimulation of the urethral sponge in particular can be a focal point for sexual arousal and orgasm.

3-31 The uterus is thought of as a passive organ which lies useless except during pregnancy and childbirth. During sexual arousal, however, its lining becomes swollen with blood and it balloons upward, enlarging the vagina. Some women actually feel it contract pleasurably.

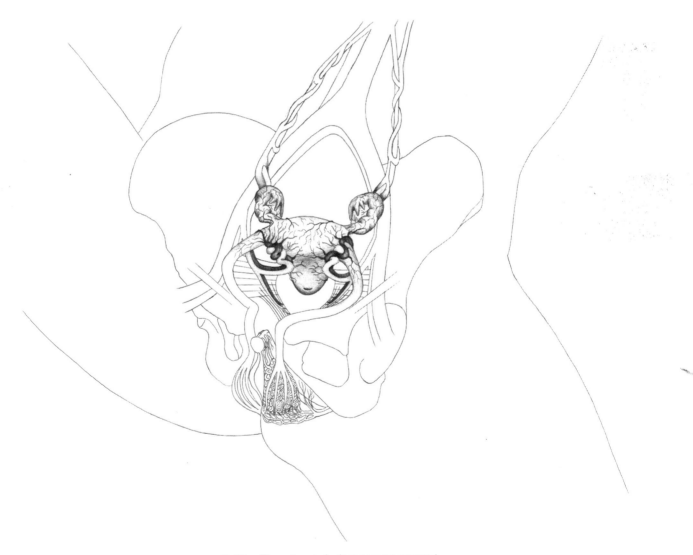

3-31   The uterus during sexual arousal

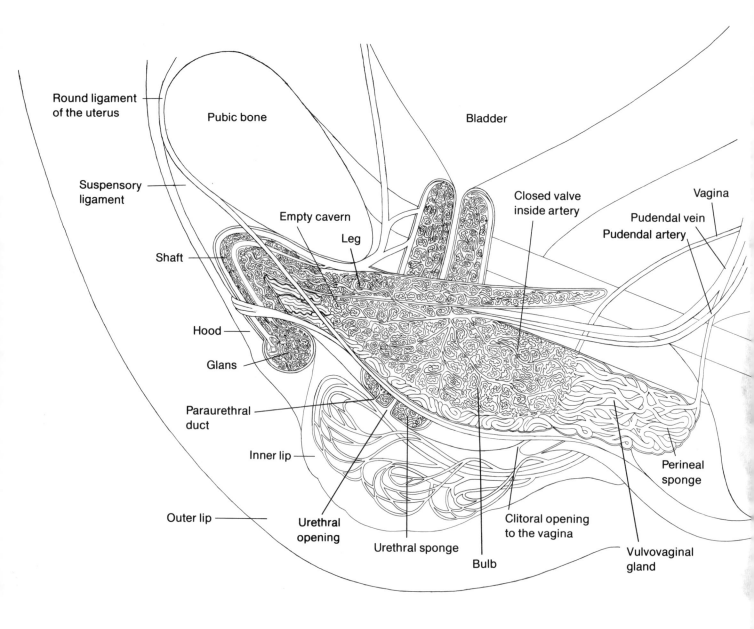

3–32 A cross section of the nonerect clitoris

3–32 The clitoris, greatly magnified, in its nonerect state. The intricate maze, created by the blood vessels and capillaries in the tissues of the glans, shaft and legs, is called corpus cavernosum, which literally means body of caverns. The urethral sponge, perineal sponge and bulbs differ from corpus cavernosum in that they are made up of tissue that is more elastic and does not become as hard during erection. This tissue is called corpus spongiosum. In the nonerect state, the valves of the clitoral arteries are closed and the valves of the veins are open.

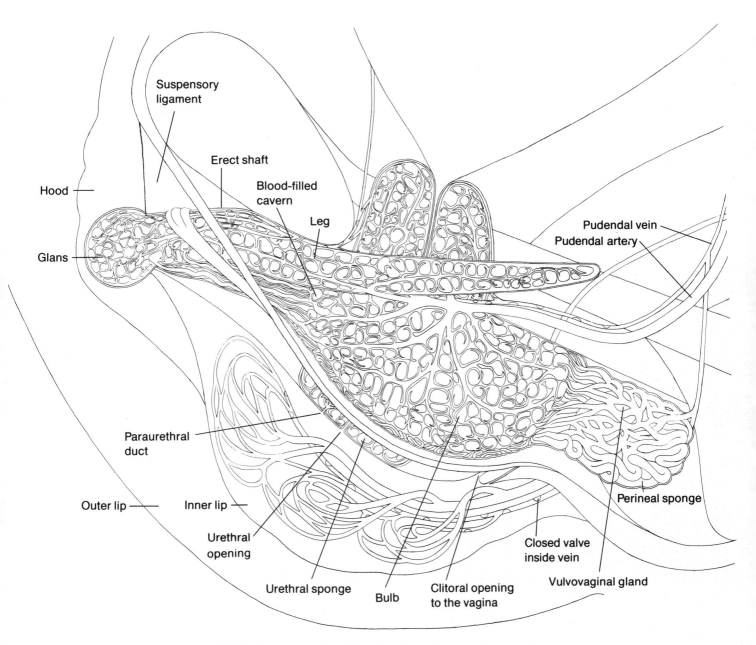

Suspensory ligament

Erect shaft

Blood-filled cavern

Leg

Hood

Glans

Pudendal vein
Pudendal artery

Paraurethral duct

Outer lip

Inner lip

Perineal sponge

Urethral opening

Urethral sponge

Bulb

Clitoral opening to the vagina

Closed valve inside vein

Vulvovaginal gland

3–33 A cross section of the clitoris during sexual arousal

3-33 During sexual arousal, the intricate chambers of these tissues fill with blood which is then trapped by valves, and the entire clitoris enlarges and changes dramatically. The glans and shaft become erect and maintain their positions until resolution. Underneath, the muscles are taut and contract in response to sexual stimulation.

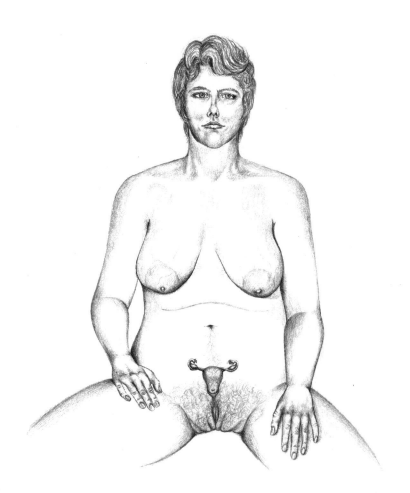

4–1   A seated woman with her uterus visible

4. A Woman's Reproductive Anatomy

Our reproductive organs include the breasts, ovaries, egg tube, uterus and vagina. The capacity of these organs to produce and nurture a ripe egg, to facilitate the union of sperm and egg, to nourish and house the developing fetus and even to provide the food for the infant's first months of life is positively dazzling and sets us apart from men. As impressive as this capacity is, however, some people tend to ignore their other equally impressive functions—which occur day in and day out throughout our entire lives These include sexual response and the manufacture and secretion of hormones. All in all, these organs play a vital role in our general health and, conversely, our health directly affects the functioning of our reproductive organs.

It is easy to get the impression from looking at these matter-of-fact illustrations that there is a scientific certainty about the menstrual cycle that does not, in fact, exist. Biologists can accurately describe the changes that take place during the menstrual cycle, but their explanations of *why* these changes take place are based on untested theories. Tragically, doctors prescribe powerful hormone-like drugs to alter the menstrual cycle without any idea of the full consequences. What this amounts to is off-the-cuff experimentation based upon an inadequate understanding of what hormones are and how they work in our bodies.

Prior to doing self-examination, most of us shared the common notion that our reproductive organs lay passively inside our bodies waiting for a sperm to come along. Or if not, we only thought of our reproductive organs when some of us occasionally became painfully aware of our uteruses during menstruation.

Feeling the dimensions of other uteruses in self-help groups, charting our cycles and becoming familiar with that whole region of our bodies gave us a practical knowledge of ourselves.

4-1 This illustration uses the see-through method to show the location of the uterus, egg tubes (fallopian tubes) and ovaries in the pelvis. One of the practical, exciting results of self-help is that participating women no longer feel embarrassed by the appearance of their bodies. High-fashion magazines and soft-porn publications on sale at every newsstand have set a standard for women: thin, hairless and unblemished. As if this weren't enough, the medical profession, looking through its disease-oriented lens, makes women feel shame and uneasiness about their reproductive organs. Minor variations, such as a tipped uterus, uneven breasts, irregular periods, even hairiness, make a woman a candidate for expensive and frequently dangerous treatment. Self-help has encouraged women to reject suggestions that these conditions are illnesses, and has returned the term "range of normal" to its true meaning, which includes all women who do not have some debilitating disease or physically uncomfortable condition.

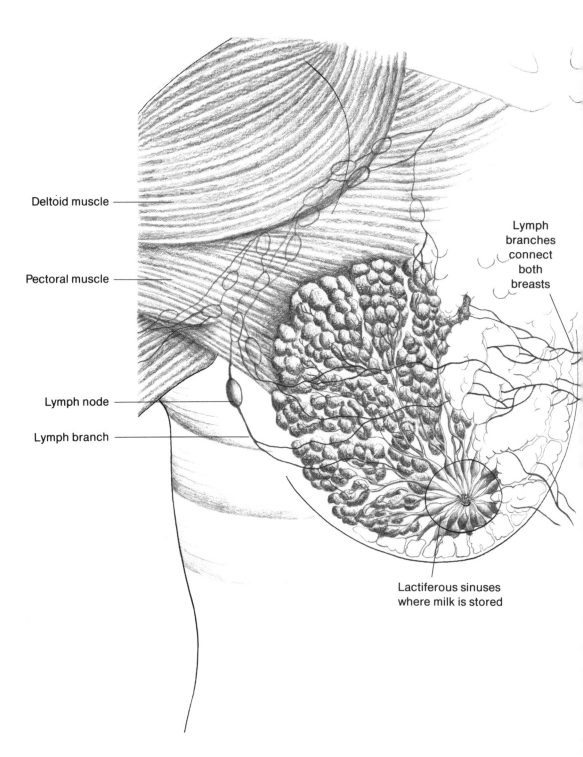

Deltoid muscle

Pectoral muscle

Lymph node

Lymph branch

Lymph
branches
connect
both
breasts

Lactiferous sinuses
where milk is stored

4–2 An inner view of a woman's breast

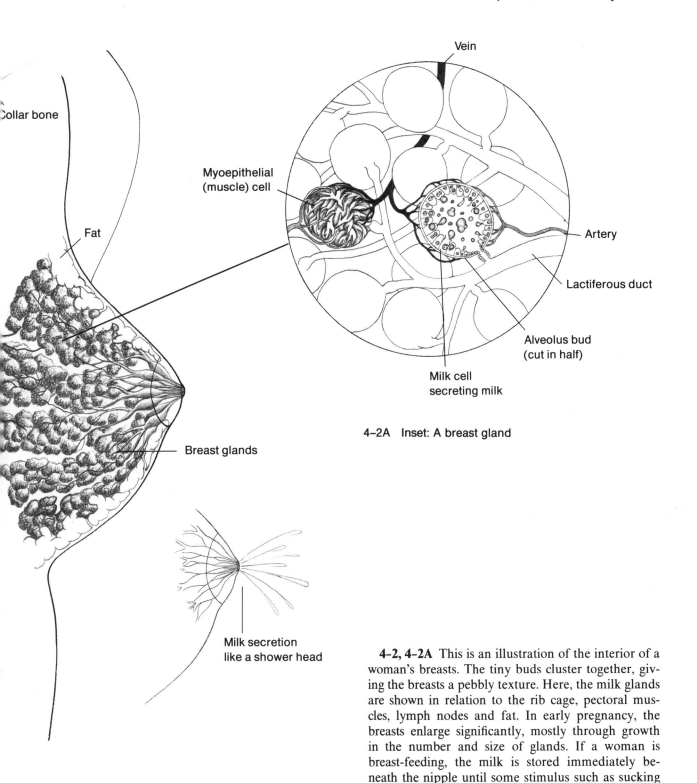

Vein

Myoepithelial
(muscle) cell

Collar bone

Fat

Artery

Lactiferous duct

Alveolus bud
(cut in half)

Milk cell
secreting milk

Breast glands

4–2A   Inset: A breast gland

Milk secretion
like a shower head

4-2, 4-2A This is an illustration of the interior of a woman's breasts. The tiny buds cluster together, giving the breasts a pebbly texture. Here, the milk glands are shown in relation to the rib cage, pectoral muscles, lymph nodes and fat. In early pregnancy, the breasts enlarge significantly, mostly through growth in the number and size of glands. If a woman is breast-feeding, the milk is stored immediately beneath the nipple until some stimulus such as sucking causes it to be squirted out. Each milk cavity has its own opening, so that the milk comes out like water from a shower head. The inset shows the muscle cells which contract during breast feeding, forcing the milk out.

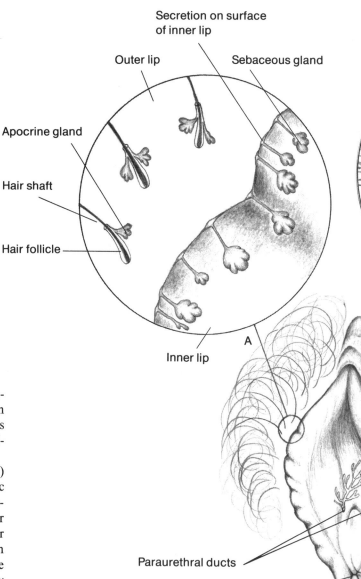

Secretion on surface
of inner lip

Outer lip

Sebaceous gland

Apocrine gland

Hair shaft

Hair follicle

Inner lip

A

Paraurethral ducts

Clitoral opening
to the vagina

Vulvovaginal glands

4-3 This rendition of secretions of the clitoris, vagina and uterus illustrates the scenting, lubrication and cleansing of the vulva and vagina. The circles show magnified areas from different parts of the genital tract.

a. Edge of the inner lip of the clitoris. Oil glands (1) are located all over the body, including the pubic mound and outer and inner lips. Other glands (2) produce sweat, though not the sweat caused by heat or exertion. It is a milky fluid which oozes from the hair follicles under conditions of excitement, stress, pain or fear. Many of them are located at the base of the hair follicles on the pubic mound and outer lips. They are called "scent" glands, since their fluid is the key ingredient needed for the formation of human odor.

b. These cells are being shed from the vaginal wall. They mix with the vaginal secretions and cause them to be cloudy.

c. Other glands, sometimes called crypts, form the passages and recesses in the cervical canal. The cells of their lining secrete clear mucus which mixes with other vaginal secretions.

d. The uterine lining is shown here during menstruation, when the top layer of superficial cells is carried out with the menstrual flow.

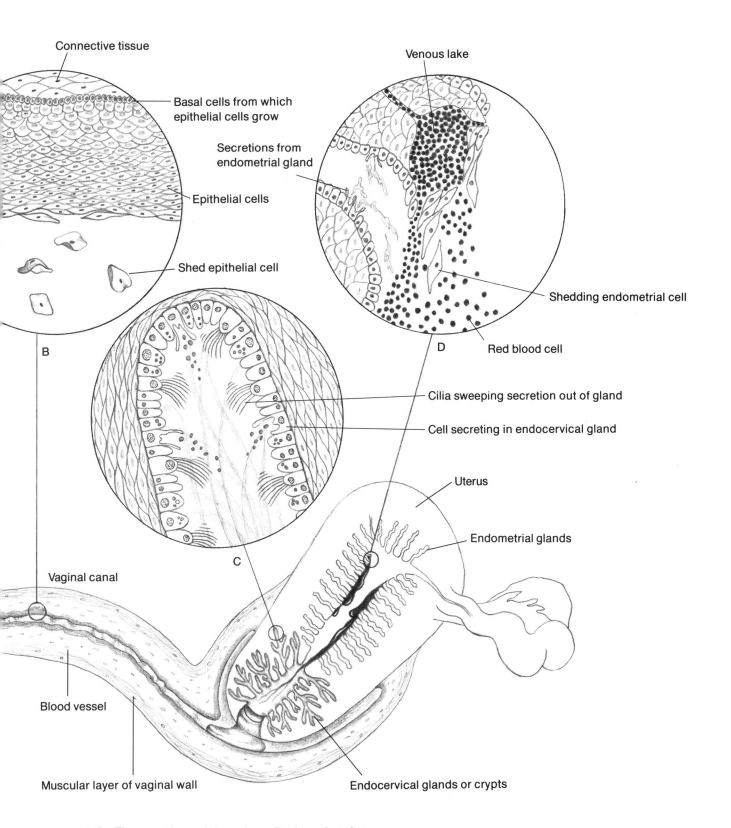

Connective tissue

Basal cells from which epithelial cells grow

Secretions from endometrial gland

Epithelial cells

Shed epithelial cell

B

Venous lake

Shedding endometrial cell

Red blood cell

D

Cilia sweeping secretion out of gland

Cell secreting in endocervical gland

Uterus

Endometrial glands

C

Vaginal canal

Blood vessel

Muscular layer of vaginal wall

Endocervical glands or crypts

4–3   The secretions of the vulva, clitoris and vagina

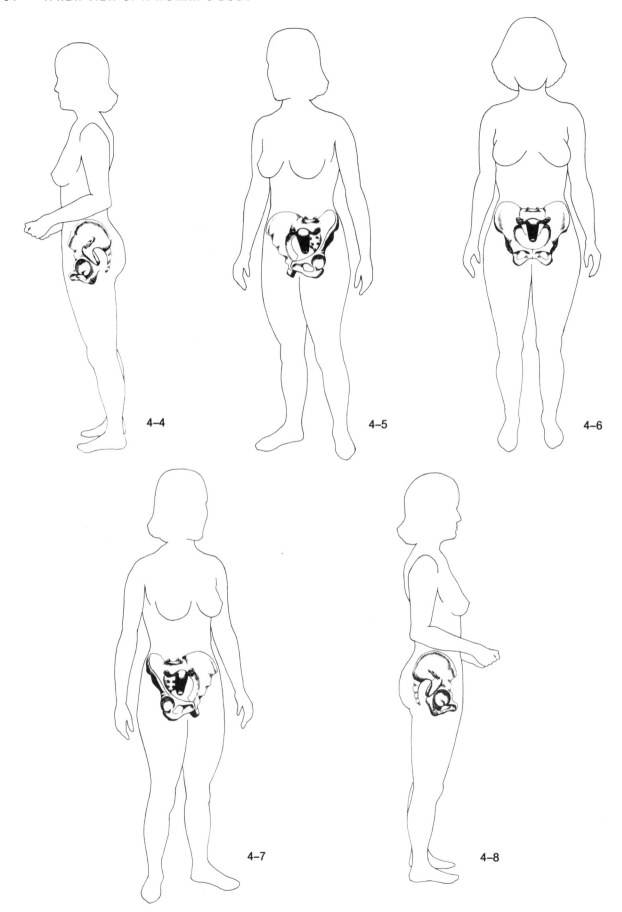

4–4

4–5

4–6

4–7

4–8

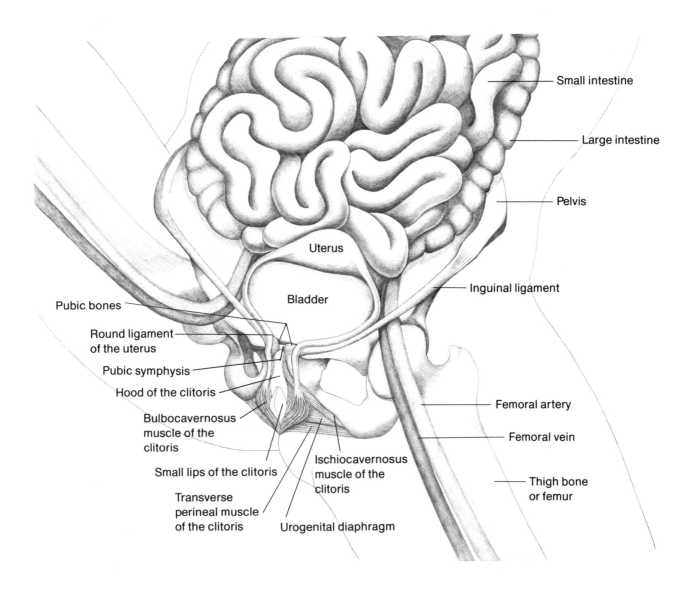

Small intestine

Large intestine

Pelvis

Uterus

Inguinal ligament

Bladder

Pubic bones

Round ligament
of the uterus

Pubic symphysis

Hood of the clitoris

Bulbocavernosus
muscle of the
clitoris

Small lips of the clitoris

Transverse
perineal muscle
of the clitoris

Ischiocavernosus
muscle of the
clitoris

Urogenital diaphragm

Femoral artery

Femoral vein

Thigh bone
or femur

4–9 A view of the uterus, intestines and bladder

4–4 to 4–8 These illustrations show the position of the pelvic bones, the position of the uterus in the pelvic cavity and their relation to the rest of the body.

4–9 In the pelvic area, the intestines rest on the uterus and bladder, which in this picture is full.

4-10 With the intestines not shown, it is possible to see the ovaries and egg tubes. In this drawing, the broad ligament covers the bladder and partially obscures the uterus. The ovaries are the most dynamic organs in a woman's body. Throughout a woman's life, from birth to death, the ovaries (and the adrenal glands) produce hormones—estrogens, androgens and progestogens. Estrogens maintain healthy skin, mucous membranes and other tissues, and, in women, produce changes in the uterus, tubes, ovaries, breasts and vagina. Androgens, mistakenly labeled "male" hormones, contribute to the growth of muscles, hair and bones. Progestogens, in women, promote the growth of the uterine lining. From the first stages of puberty, on a more or less regular basis, the ovaries undergo radical changes during the menstrual cycle that culminate when a ripe egg slowly emerges from the ovarian wall and travels down the egg tube into the uterus.

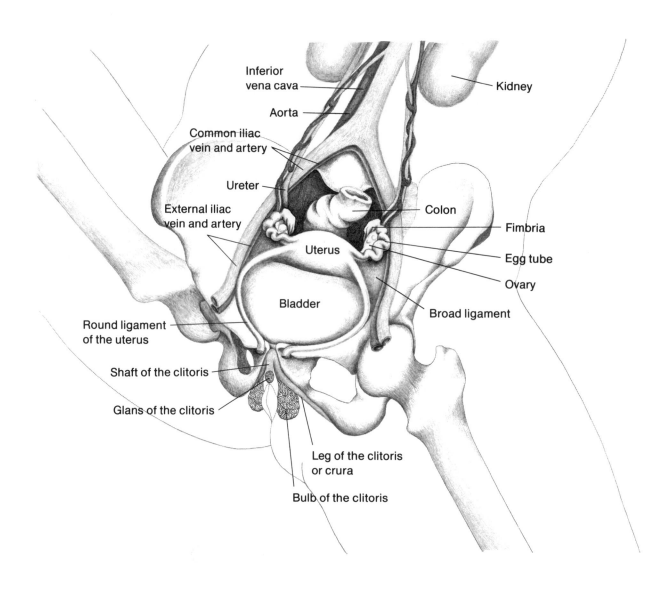

4-10   A view of the uterus and bladder with the intestines not shown

The 28-day cycle is a medical myth. Although most women have approximately monthly cycles, healthy and fertile women can have cycles as infrequently as two or three times a year. Women can miss their periods, have extra periods or have more bleeding or less bleeding during their periods, due to stress or nutritional deficiencies. It is very typical for a woman's period to be delayed anywhere from three months to a year and a half after she discontinues the Pill. Most women produce eggs regularly, somewhere between 21 and 45 days. Other women have very long cycles and ovulate, it is believed, about two weeks before menstruation begins. However, in many cycles, no egg is produced and on occasion women ovulate more than once in an otherwise ordinary cycle.

4-11 The uterus, a powerful muscular organ, is suspended in the pelvis by ligaments. They provide support, but allow for uterine movement or growth within the pelvis. In this illustration, the intestines and bladder are not shown.

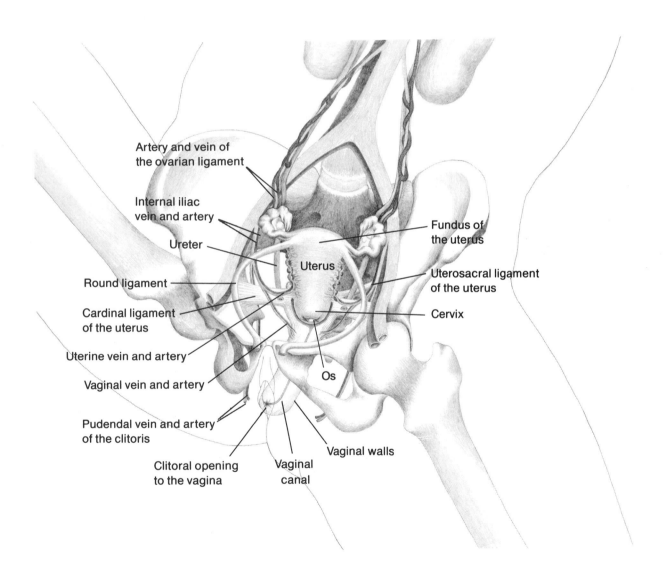

4-11   A view of the uterus with the intestines and bladder not shown

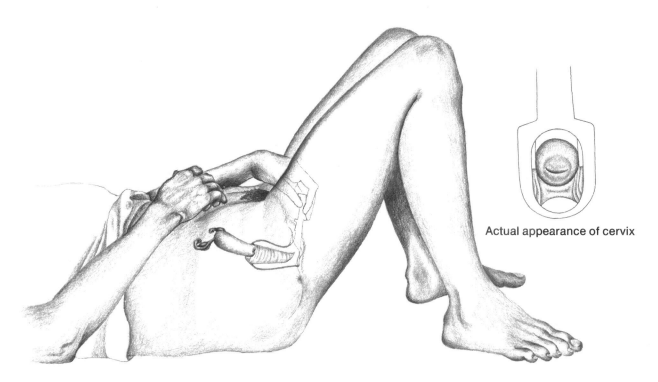

Actual appearance of cervix

4–12   A woman with a tipped-up uterus doing self-examination

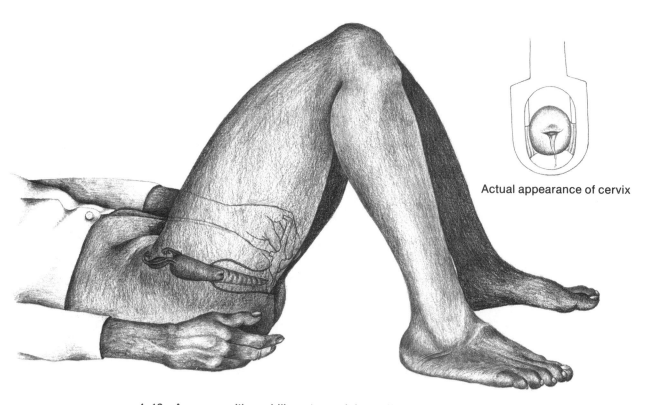

Actual appearance of cervix

4–13   A woman with a midline uterus doing self-examination

4-12 Women whose uteruses are not front and center are told that they have "tipped uteruses," usually with the implication that this is abnormal. On the contrary, every woman's uterus is tipped one way or another, whether it is forward (anteverted), middle or back (retroverted). Indeed, the uterus can change positions and it has a tendency to retreat when touched. This woman's uterus is tipped up slightly.

4-13 If a woman is not pregnant, her uterus is about three or four inches long, slightly elongated and has a mucous membrane lining that grows and sheds in the course of her menstrual cycle. The egg tubes and ovaries are attached to the top, called the fundus. Here, the uterus is lying flat, in a midline position.

4-14 Far from passive, the muscular structure of the uterus contracts in response to sexual stimulation and at the moment of orgasm, and in response to menstruation and breast-feeding, dilation of the cervix or manual stimulation. This woman's uterus is tipped downward.

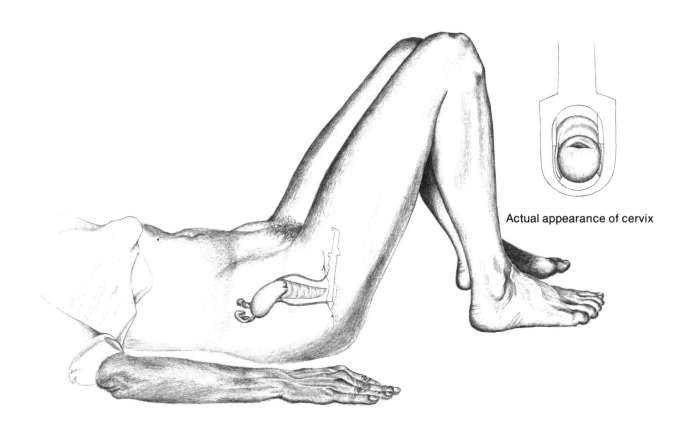

Actual appearance of cervix

4-14   A woman with a tipped-back uterus doing self-examination

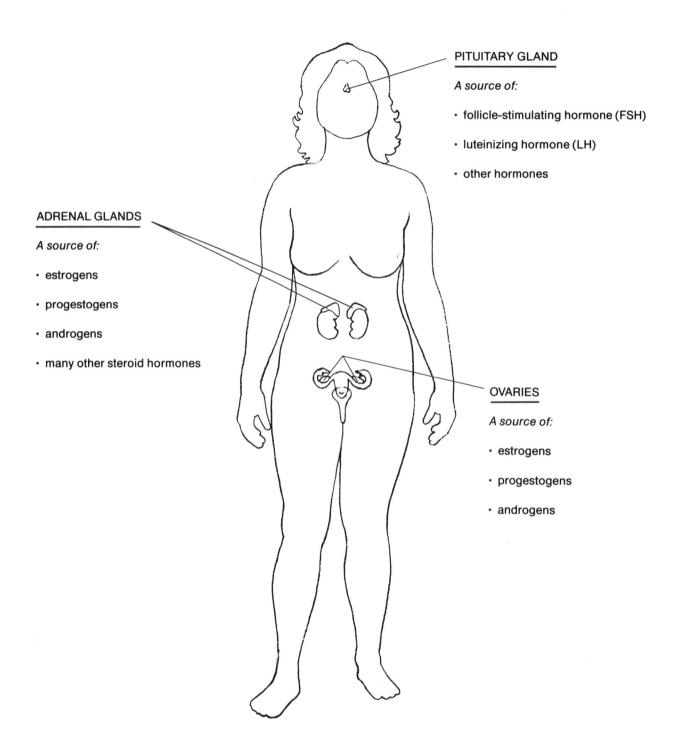

PITUITARY GLAND

A source of:

• follicle-stimulating hormone (FSH)

• luteinizing hormone (LH)

• other hormones

ADRENAL GLANDS

A source of:

• estrogens

• progestogens

• androgens

• many other steroid hormones

OVARIES

A source of:

• estrogens

• progestogens

• androgens

4–15   The glands which secrete hormones: The endocrine glands

4-15 Hormones are incredibly minute substances that are manufactured in certain glands and travel through the bloodstream; they exert specific influences (and sometimes cause dramatic changes) in other parts of the body. Simplistically speaking, clinicians often view hormones as illusive forces over which we have no control. The attention that has been devoted to understanding their sources and functions has been focused almost exclusively upon their role in sexual maturation and reproduction, and the vital part hormones play in everyday health has often been overlooked.

Hormones are thought of in terms of some sort of magical "balance," and people who study hormones, called endocrinologists, have developed an elaborate theory to explain the fact that the body constantly readjusts hormones levels.

This theory suggests that a woman's body works like a thermostat, turning on and off throughout the menstrual cycle to control the ebb and flow of hormones in order to maintain that balance. The theory also assumes that only certain parts of the body are affected by hormones.

Some dissident scientists have pointed out the flaws in the theory. First, it does not take into account any external influences, such as stress, exercise and nutrition; nor does it allow for unexpected changes in hormone levels. In addition, it does not take into account recent information on the influential role of vitamins in the hormone cycle.

No one has ever seen a hormone, but it is possible to measure in the laboratory levels of hormones in the blood at a given time. It is thought that before a woman ovulates, FSH (follicle-stimulating hormone) and LH (luteinizing hormone) are released by the pituitary into the bloodstream. Endocrinologists believe that these two hormones play a major role in the development of the egg sac or follicle (described in this chapter on page 72) from which the egg pops (hence, the name "follicle-stimulating" hormone).

When the follicle begins to develop, blood levels of estrogen rise significantly, as compared to other times in the cycle.

After ovulation, when the yellow body or corpus luteum (also described on page 72) develops, progesterone levels appear to be high, suggesting, perhaps, that the corpus luteum is a major producer of progesterone.

Research has found that just before menstruation, blood levels of estrogen and progesterone are lower, though the exact relationship between blood hormone levels and menstruation is not known (although it is assumed to be significant).

Endocrinology is an infant science; there is only a small amount of scientifically proven data, and most of that information has come from studying women who have sought medical help because of disease. It seems safer to us to observe what seems to occur than to construct theories and try to fit small bits of data into them.

Many women are unaware of the dynamic events of ovulation unless they experience *Mittelschmerz*, the pain that occurs on alternate sides of the pelvic area every other cycle when the egg passes through the ovarian wall. Many women feel no sensation at all as the egg bursts forth and begins its several-days' journey down the egg tube and, if it does not meet a sperm, into the uterus and out with the menstrual flow.

The ovaries are two endocrine glands about the size of unshelled almonds (about one to one-and-a-half inches) which contain as many as 450,000 eggs, dispense one or occasionally two eggs on a regular basis, and manufacture hormones.

At various points in the menstrual cycle, the ovarian cells actually develop new structures, the follicles and the corpus luteum, as the ovary releases an egg and repairs itself. If one ovary is removed, the one remaining will take over and ovulate every cycle.

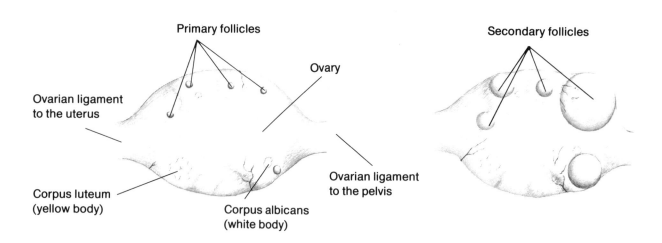

4–16   The ovary with primary follicles

4–17   The ovary with secondary follicles

4-16 Prior to ovulation, a crop of follicles begins to develop. Each one consists of an egg surrounded by a layer of grainy cells. These primary follicles are shown as they appear five days to a week prior to ovulation. Shown in this drawing is an old yellow body (corpus luteum) from a previous ovulation, now called a white body, shrinking back into the ovary, and old primary follicles (sacs) which never fully developed. These follicles, referred to as atretic, also gradually shrink back into the body of the ovary.

4-17 In the next couple of days, about 20 of the primary follicles will continue to develop and enlarge. The grainy cells duplicate, causing the follicle wall to thicken, and the egg floats in a gelatin-like mass. One or more of these follicles, now called secondary follicles, grows larger than the rest and bulges toward the outer surface of the ovary, forming a bump. The secondary follicles in this drawing are as they appear two days before ovulation.

4-18 As ovulation approaches, the ovary becomes enlarged with blood and the ligaments contract, pulling the ovary closer toward the uterus. One of the follicles, now called a tertiary follicle, often grows to half the size of the ovary.

4-19 At the moment of ovulation, the tertiary folli-cle wall ruptures and the egg, embedded in a glob of jellylike matter and blood, oozes out. Some women feel this as a sharp pain, some a dull ache and some do not feel it at all.

4-20 The egg tubes are soft and flexible. They open above each ovary like a canopy with a tapered fringe. Active, hairlike projections, called cilia, cover the undersurface. The walls of the tubes are made of smooth muscle tissue and lined with folded, cilia-covered mucous membranes.

Around the time of ovulation, the blood vessels in the egg tubes become filled with blood and contrac-tions cause the fingerlike projections to curl around the ovary, brushing across the surface. The rapid beating of the cilia brings the egg in its halo of follicu-lar fluid into the tube.

4-21 The pocket formed by the ruptured follicle fills with clotted blood. The cells which make up the follicle wall begin to grow very large and fill with droplets of fat. The follicle wall (here cut away) be-comes wrinkled and fluted and begins to collapse. The follicle is now called the corpus luteum and it is thought that this structure secretes higher levels of progestogens. This view shows the thickened, folded follicular walls after the emergence of the egg.

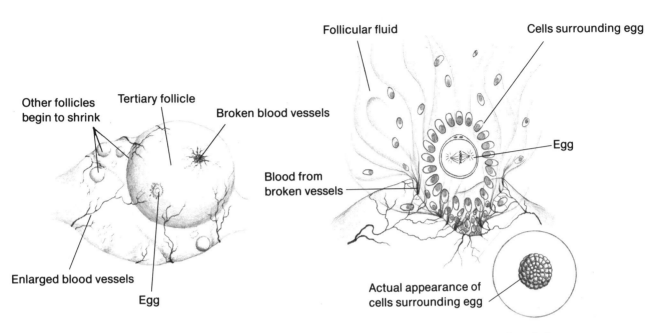

Other follicles begin to shrink

Tertiary follicle

Broken blood vessels

Enlarged blood vessels

Egg

4-18   The ovary with tertiary follicle

Follicular fluid

Cells surrounding egg

Egg

Blood from broken vessels

Actual appearance of cells surrounding egg

4-19   The ovary at the moment of ovulation

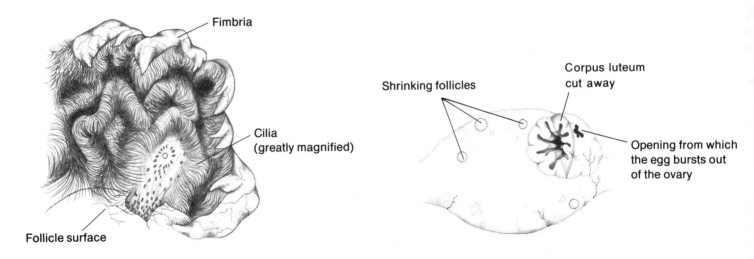

Fimbria

Cilia (greatly magnified)

Follicle surface

4-20   The opening of the egg tubes above the ovary

Shrinking follicles

Corpus luteum cut away

Opening from which the egg bursts out of the ovary

4-21   The ovary with the corpus luteum (yellow body) after ovulation

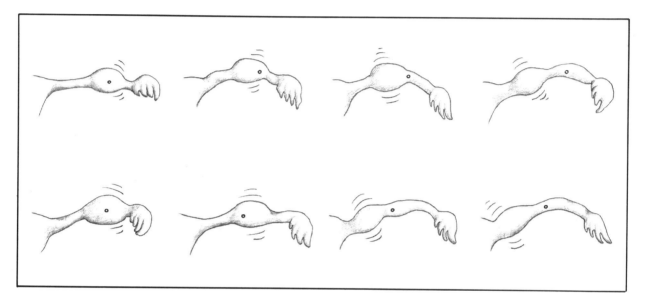

4-22   The egg tube contracting

4-22 The egg is propelled by muscular contractions halfway down the tube, where it hesitates for some unknown reason for three or four days. Then it is pushed rapidly into the uterus.

4-23 The muscular wall of the uterus in midcycle is cut away to reveal its lining. The magnified insets illustrate (from left to right) cellular changes involved in menstruation.

Following menstruation and throughout the first half of the menstrual cycle, the proliferative phase, the cells that form the endometrium reproduce, thickening the lining of the uterus.

a. After ovulation occurs, glands on the surface of the uterine lining secrete mucus which comes from the single layer of cells which lines each gland. This is called the secretory phase of a woman's menstrual cycle.

b. A few hours before the flow begins, the spiral arteries of the lining (the endometrium) constrict, cutting off the blood supply to its surface. The blood near the surface pools in pockets called venous lakes, and cells begin to die for lack of oxygen. When they are full, the venous lakes burst, and blood and dead cells from the surface of the lining form the menstrual flow. The lining begins to shrink from this loss of blood and other fluid.

c. During menstruation, the lining does not shed entirely. The bottom layer of cells remains, starting to grow again immediately. It will become the top layer of cells to be shed during the next cycle.

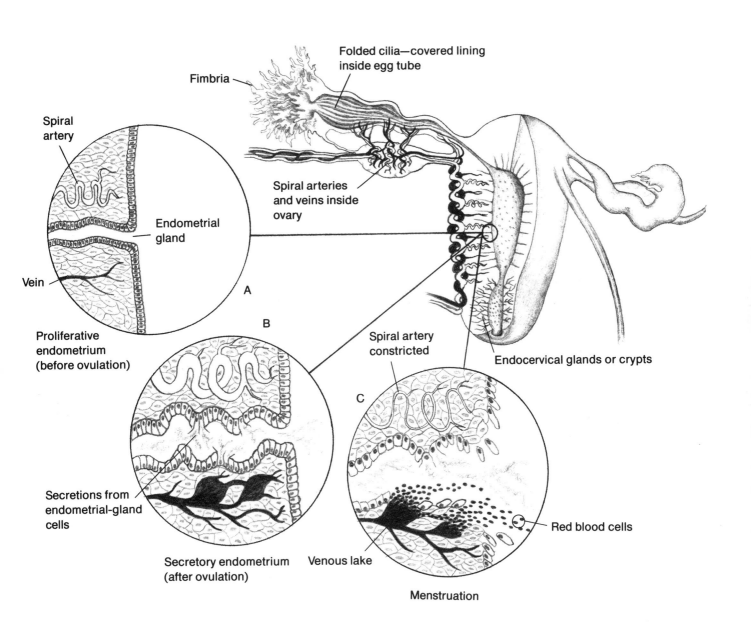

Folded cilia—covered lining
inside egg tube

Fimbria

Spiral
artery

Spiral arteries
and veins inside
ovary

Endometrial
gland

Vein

A

Proliferative
endometrium
(before ovulation)

B

Spiral artery
constricted

Endocervical glands or crypts

C

Secretions from
endometrial-gland
cells

Red blood cells

Secretory endometrium
(after ovulation)

Venous lake

Menstruation

4-23   The lining of the uterus

Menopause

The prevailing attitude of the medical profession toward menopause is that it is an illness. Hot flashes, depression, insomnia, fatigue or a dry vagina are thought to be due to a slowing down of the ovaries and, therefore, are treated with hormone-like drugs.

When women seek information about menopause, they often encounter a number of common myths:

- that the ovaries stop functioning and a woman is infertile;
- that a woman has an estrogen deficiency and, hence, a hormone imbalance;
- that a woman gains weight and her bones become brittle;
- that estrogen replacement therapy (ERT) will correct problems associated with menopause.

There is no scientific proof for any of the above suppositions! In fact,

- a healthy woman's ovaries function throughout her life and continue to produce hormones and, less often after menopause, eggs;
- a woman frequently has higher estrogen levels *after* her periods cease, and there is no ideal balance to be disturbed;
- androgens, which influence the libido or interest in sex, continue to be produced and, in many women, tend to be higher after menopause;
- estrogen replacement therapy can, at best, temporarily mask the symptoms blamed on menopause. At worst, by suppressing ovarian activity, it can cause the ovary to atrophy and also increase a woman's risk of cancer.

With regard to menopause, doctors never talk about the aging process. Highly regarded hormonal specialists, however, know that the severe symptoms blamed on menopause are due to the aging process or, even more likely, to lack of exercise, an inactive sex life, constant stress, ill health or vitamin deficiencies. We are made to think that it is beyond our power to correct these problems without medication. In truth, efforts made to change diet and to increase exercise are richly rewarded with improved health, more energy, a toned body and elimination of so-called menopausal symptoms.

Women do ovulate after menopause, but much less frequently than before. Fertility is, after all, dependent upon other factors besides ovulation: particularly the availability of a healthy, fertile partner and an active sex life. In addition, there are a host of identifiable outside influences, such as cigarettes and alcohol, the Pill, tranquilizers, poor nutrition, poor circulation, a poorly functioning thyroid or liver damage, which can affect the ovaries and hormones adversely.

The symptom most often associated with menopause is the hot flash which is also symptomatic of hypoglycemia (low blood sugar), a condition which affects a significant percentage of the population. A dry vagina, another frequent symptom, is also very common among women who do not have frequent sex. And the loss of a sense of well-being or depression is a widespread phenomenon among people in their middle years.

Hot flashes, or hot flushes, are uncomfortable, inconvenient and sometimes frightening to many women. A feeling of warmth all over, disorientation, tingling in the hands and feet, insomnia, nervousness and headaches are sensations that many women experience. Many say that they tend to sweat profusely during and after a hot flash. (Sweating is the body's attempt to cool itself and is a natural reaction to heat.)

While hot flashes are disconcerting, they are not dangerous. Some women choose to live with them until they go away, instead of taking hormone-like drugs, and try instead to do strenuous exercises and to improve their nutrition. Women who have infrequent opportunities for sex have found that masturbating often increases vaginal lubrication.

If you have a tendency to have a tender or dry vagina, some home remedies can be soothing and can help make sexual intercourse more comfortable. Aloe vera gel, yogurt or the kinds of ointments used for diaper rash applied to the skin are often helpful. Unless you have an infection, douching is one of the worst things to do; it robs the mucous membranes of any natural lubrication they have. Likewise, using so-called "feminine deodorants," which contain harsh chemicals and alcohols, can intensify a tendency toward dryness. Tight-fitting pants can also make matters worse and encourage infection by preventing air from circulating and adding stress to tender tissues.

Estrogen Replacement Therapy

If menopausal symptoms are not caused by a lack of estrogen, then why do physicians prescribe estrogen replacement therapy?

Women do notice dramatic changes when they take hormone-like drugs. The drugs "pump up" cells, causing them to retain water. This can make wrinkles less apparent, the mucous membranes of the vagina more supple, and increased cellular activity can create a sense of well-being and more energy. These "bene-fits," however, disappear when you stop taking the drugs.

The hormone-like drugs used for ERT are similar to those in the Pill and have no chemical relation to the natural estrogen in a woman's body. They are manufactured from either coal tar or from a concoction of chemicals and mare's urine. They are especially inappropriate for women who have kidney disease, epilepsy, depression or liver disease. Even healthy women who take ERT are subject to a substantially higher risk—almost 15 percent higher—of cancer of the uterine lining. And these drugs actually suppress the activity of the ovaries, thus medically inducing atrophy—a sort of death—of the ovaries.

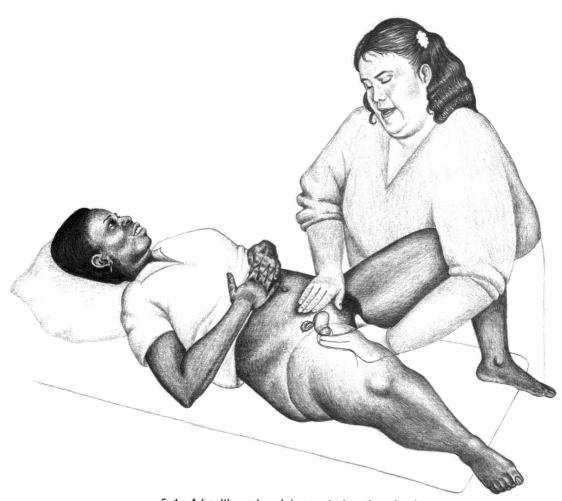

5–1 A health worker doing a uterine size check

5 · A Well-Woman Exam

The well-woman examination, done in a clinic or doctor's office, focuses on maintenance of the health of the sexual and reproductive organs, routine screening tests, identification and treatment of common conditions, determination of pregnancy and birth control services.

Combined with the taking of a careful health history, an examination of the vulva and vagina, cervix, uterus, tubes and ovaries is useful for identifying anything unusual which might indicate a problem or a condition hidden from view.

5-1 A uterine check can be done by a trained health worker or nurse, but in most doctors' offices, the pelvic exam is always done by the doctor. If the uterus is difficult to feel because it is "tipped," the physician often does a rectovaginal exam. This exam is done by inserting the index finger into the vagina and the middle finger into the rectum, then pressing down fairly hard on the abdomen above the pubic hairline. Unlike the uterine size check, which should not hurt, the rectovaginal exam is definitely uncomfortable, so it is important for the doctor to ask your permission beforehand.

Women usually avoid the gynecologist's office unless they have to go for treatment of a bothersome infection or identification of a suspected problem. Many women prefer going to a clinic or, if possible, to a nontraditional women's clinic where there is an emphasis on health education and sharing of information.

In a traditional physician's office, services tend to be rendered in an officious, formal fashion and women are expected to be passive and, for the most part, unquestioning.

The exam ritual, which varies little from office to office and seems peculiar to doctors trained in the United States, creates a distance between the doctor and the woman seeking health care. Some people feel that it actually only serves the convenience of the physicians. The drape, for example, prevents a woman from seeing what is going on. When one really stops to question this seemingly considerate gesture, it is clear that it inhibits the flow of information and allows the doctor to work undisturbed (which would be okay if he or she were working on a car instead of on your body).

The standard, but most uncomfortable, and, for many women, humiliating part of the exam routine is the requirement that a woman put her feet in stirrups and have her buttocks half off the end of the table. This custom arises from the physician's insistence on having the speculum handle pointed down—slightly more convenient for the doctor and a *lot* more uncomfortable for you. Neither a uterine check nor a speculum exam requires the use of stirrups.

It is also customary in most doctor's offices for a female nurse to be present at all exams to act as a buffer between you and the doctor to make sure no improprieties occur. This custom is a tacit acknowledgment of the reality that feminists have exposed:

79

that a male doctor putting on a white coat does not change his socialization or attitudes toward women.

Self-helpers have found through experience in dealing with doctors and hospitals that knowing their rights and being assertive can provide access to information and, hence, better health care.

Through legislation and court decisions, patients have gained the right to participate actively in their treatment. In many states, everyone who goes to a doctor has the right to

- read her own medical charts and records;
- have a full explanation of all examinations;
- ask questions about cost, office routines and payment;
- receive treatment without the consent of a spouse or parent;
- read all literature accompanying medication.

One way to assure that you have these rights is to take a patient advocate, who may be a medically trained person or a friend, with you when you go to a clinic or doctor's office for an examination, particularly if any type of treatment is anticipated. An advocate has nothing to gain or lose and can question the doctor or staff in a way that you might not feel free to do. The advocate can question, support you and help you weigh information and make decisions.

Self-helpers have found it helpful in relating to a doctor to be fully dressed when meeting her or him for the first time, or at least to be sitting up when the doctor enters the room. It's also a good idea to shake hands, and, if you are addressed by your first name, you should feel free to address the doctor on a first-name basis also.

5-2 to 5-5 Although the Pap smear is generally thought of as a test for cancer of the cervix, it also

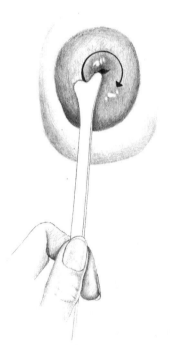

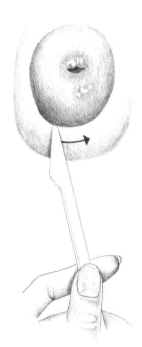

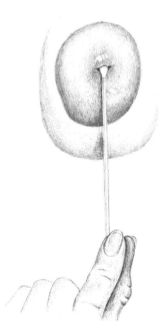

5-2 Pap smear: Cells being taken from the face of the cervix

5-3 Pap smear: Cells being taken from the vagina

5-4 Pap smear: Cells being taken from the opening of the cervix

screens for vaginal conditions such as yeast, trichomonas or bacterial conditions, as well as for some conditions like dysplasia (unusual development or alteration of the size, shape or organization of cells), or cervicitis (irritation of the cervix), which can be precancerous.

It takes about 30 seconds to do a Pap smear and, if done properly, *it should not hurt.* Smears of cells are taken from three different sites and placed on a glass slide. First, they are taken from the face of the cervix by rotating the tip of a wooden spatula 360 degrees at the cervical opening. Then cells are gently scraped from the vaginal walls and secretions underneath the cervix are picked up. Finally, cells are wiped from the cervical opening with a cotton-tipped swab. The slide is then covered with a chemical fixative and sent to the laboratory for analysis. (The first three steps can be done in any order.)

The Pap smear result returns with a reading between Class I and Class V.

Class I: Cells appear normal; negative for cancer;

Class II: Atypical: cells display changes which probably are a result of infection or irritation of the vagina or cervix which may be minor; no cancerous cells present; possibly mild dysplasia.

Class IIIa: Atypical cells are present, indicating moderate dysplasia. A noncancerous but unusual development of cells; not necessarily indicative of disease. Repeat smear suggested.

Class IIIb: Cells present are suggestive of possible cancer. Biopsy suggested.

Class IV: Some cells present which are very suggestive of a small, noninvasive cancer (cancer *in situ*).

Class V: Large numbers of cells present which appear cancerous.

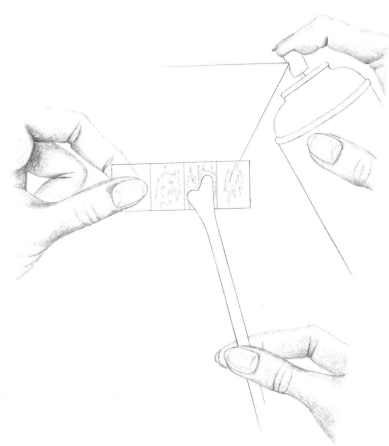

5–5 Pap smear: Spraying preservative on the pap smear slide

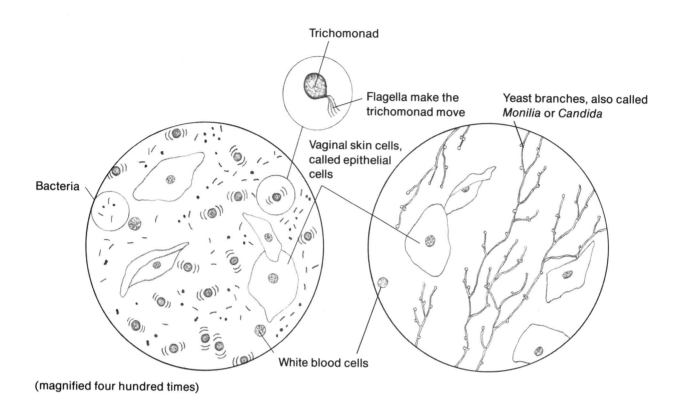

Trichomonad

Flagella make the trichomonad move

Yeast branches, also called *Monilia* or *Candida*

Vaginal skin cells, called epithelial cells

Bacteria

White blood cells

(magnified four hundred times)

5–6   Trichomonas and yeast seen through a microscope

The Pap smear also yields an indirect and *very approximate* measure of hormonal activity, called the maturation index. This measure notes the percentage of basal (bottom), parabasal (middle) and superficial (top) types of cells present. This indicates the rate at which cells from the vagina and cervix are being pushed up from the bottom to the top layers to be sloughed off from the mucous membrane lining. A higher percentage of superficial cells supposedly indicates a higher level of estrogen. (This method is quite fallible and no conclusion about a woman's overall hormonal activity should be drawn from the results of one Pap smear.)

5–6 If you suspect trichomonas, you can have a slide made from your vaginal secretions and have it looked at under a microscope. The discharge from trichomonas is yellowish or greenish, frothy and marked by an acrid odor. If trichomonads are present, these tiny one-celled organisms, which resemble tadpoles, can be seen swimming around on the slide.

Many women consult their gynecologist when they develop a white, sort of clumpy discharge which causes itching and burning and has a pungent odor—the typical symptoms of a yeast overgrowth, which doctors call an "infection" and self-helpers call a "yeast condition." To confirm the presence of yeast, a slide can be made and viewed under a microscope. You can be sure you have a yeast condition if large colonies of it are present.

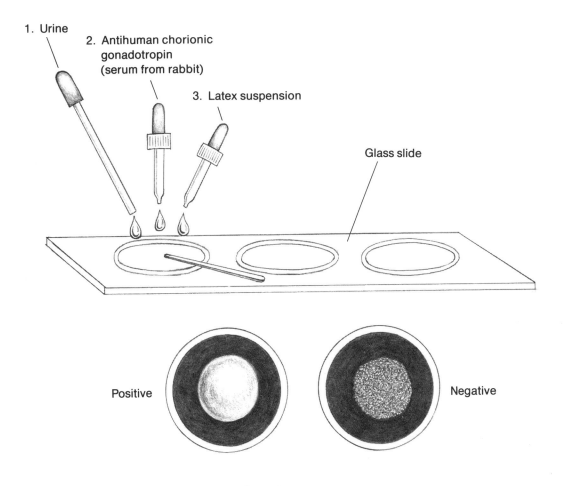

5–7   The urine pregnancy test

5–7 The widely used two-minute urine pregnancy test can be done by a woman herself and is usually sufficient to indicate if she is pregnant—if she is at least 41 days from the beginning of her last period. By this time (when she is about two weeks late), there should be enough of the pregnancy hormone in her urine to be detected chemically.

The most widely used urine pregnancy test is frequently done by women themselves in women-controlled clinics. On the slide, one drop of urine is mixed with one drop of a clear liquid which is the chemical opposite of the pregnancy hormone. A drop of an opaque latex solution makes the reaction visible. If enough hormone of pregnancy is present, it will combine with the chemical and the solution will remain smooth and creamy. If there is none, or not enough, the solution will break up and look grainy. A small proportion of women will be pregnant and still not test positive. Women occasionally have incorrect negative readings if they are taking certain types of tranquilizers or aspirin or have had large amounts of marijuana in the last 24 hours. Often this simple urine test only tells a woman what she already knows—by the time this test is valid, she is likely to have experienced one or more of the classic signs of pregnancy: tender breasts, fatigue or sleepiness, frequency of urination, missed period, changes in appetite and nausea.

A two-hour urine test on the market is similar to the test described here. Called the EPT or Early Pregnancy Test, it is available at most pharmacies. This test seems to be fairly accurate and, again, usually confirms what a woman already suspects. The major disadvantage of this test is that some women find the results difficult to interpret.

5-8 If home remedies or prescription drugs fail to clear up a cervical infection that has become bothersome, some form of cauterization can be done to remove chronically infected tissue. There are three types of cautery (burning) which are used by physicians:

a. The most frequently used form burns away tissue with an electric tool which has a looped wire or metal end. The hot metal is placed against the cervix, and often the burning is done in a star-shaped pattern. Cauterization does not hurt, but some women report that it feels "weird" and sometimes causes cramping, especially afterward, accompanied by a heavy discharge.

b. Cryosurgery, or the freezing of tissue, is also done fairly frequently. A metal cone-shaped tool hooked up to liquid nitrogen or freon is applied to the cervix at the opening. After three to five minutes, the tissue is frozen and white. In a few days, the dead cells swell up with moisture and form a bubble over the opening. As they break, the dead cells fall off and are replaced by new, healthy cells.

c. Cauterization can also be done chemically, by applying a caustic liquid with a cotton-tipped swab.

This is an older method which is not as widely used. It is, however, less traumatic to the cervix than the other two methods.

The surgical treatment for more serious conditions of the cervix is explained in Chapter 10.

5-9 A gonorrhea culture (GC) is a screening test which should be offered routinely as part of a well-woman exam. The test is only effective about half the time, so some women choose to have one every few months or whenever they are in the clinic. The test is done by inserting a cotton-tipped swab into the mouth of the cervix for about ten seconds and then wiping it on a culture plate. This picks up skin cells, secretions and any bacteria. Gonorrhea is on the rise; therefore, women who have more than one partner, or whose partners have sex with other people, have reason to be wary. Women usually have no symptoms until the disease is in an advanced stage and permanent damage may have occurred. Although lesbians tend to have fewer venereal diseases than heterosexual women, they also can pick up infections, including gonorrhea, from a sexual partner.

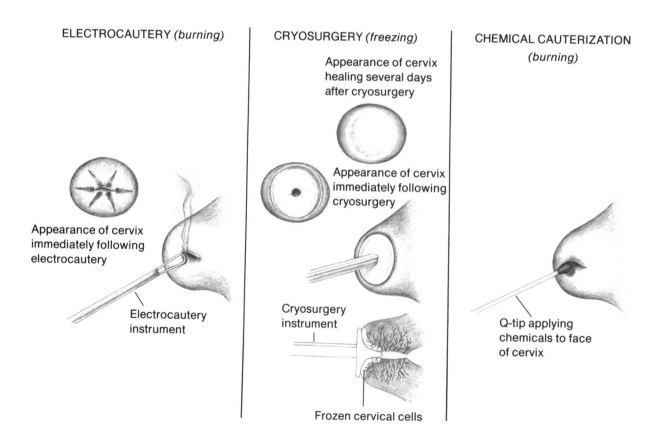

ELECTROCAUTERY *(burning)*

Appearance of cervix immediately following electrocautery

Electrocautery instrument

CRYOSURGERY *(freezing)*

Appearance of cervix healing several days after cryosurgery

Appearance of cervix immediately following cryosurgery

Cryosurgery instrument

Frozen cervical cells

CHEMICAL CAUTERIZATION *(burning)*

Q-tip applying chemicals to face of cervix

5–8 The techniques of cervical cauterization

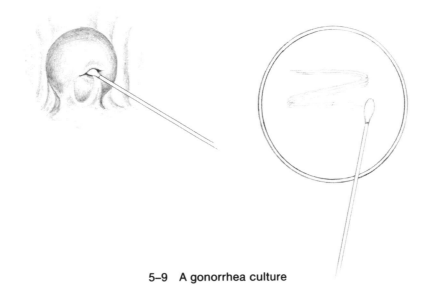

5–9   A gonorrhea culture

5-10 More and more women are seeking out gynecologists and clinics who will perform artificial insemination. Women who do not have partners, women whose partners are sterile, or lesbians can become pregnant by having semen from a donor placed in their vaginas. This procedure might, in fact, be more appropriately called "donor insemination," since "artificial insemination" sounds so technical. Actually, this procedure is very simple—so simple, in fact, that some women do it in their homes, entirely outside of a medical setting.

In the doctor's office or clinic, semen, which is usually acquired from a cryobank (which houses frozen tissues), is inserted into a woman's vagina by means of a syringe or a strawlike container. Sometimes a diaphragm is used to hold the semen near the cervix.

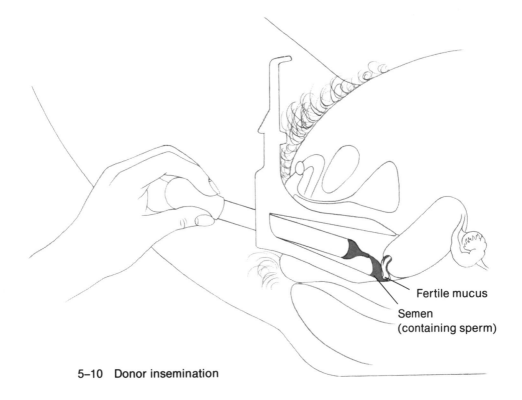

Fertile mucus

Semen
(containing sperm)

5–10   Donor insemination

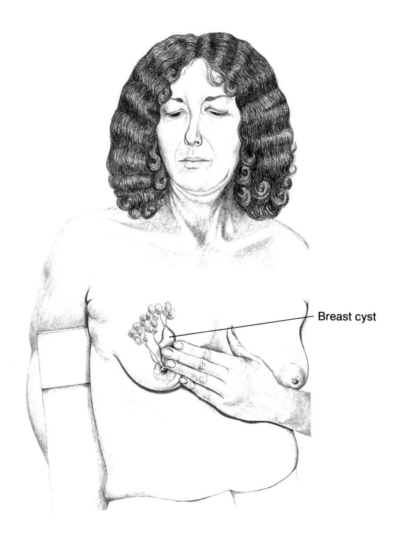

Breast cyst

6-1   A woman feeling a breast cyst

6 · Universal Health Problems of Women

Before self-help revived traditional healing practices, women had to rely on their doctors to treat minor but annoying conditions such as overgrowths of yeast, urinary tract infections, hemorrhoids, menstrual cramps, fibrous growths of the uterus and chronic irritations of the cervix. Drugs or surgery are the standard medical treatment for all of these conditions. The standard self-help approach is everyday common sense and home remedies or over-the-counter preparations which work *just as well or better* than heavy drugs or surgical procedures in many instances. Indeed, the medical profession has not been particularly interested in some of the more common problems of women, and consequently has little to offer. Physicians are typically uninterested in exercise and nutrition or in environmental factors which affect women's health. Women often need to change not only their course of treatment, but also significant factors in their life styles before they can permanently remedy some chronic problems.

Sharing self-help information gives women practical, nonmedical alternatives for dealing with everyday health problems. It is essential, however, to know when home remedies are appropriate and when to seek medical help. The more information a woman has, the more comfortable she is about a decision to treat herself. If she decides to see a doctor, having good information also helps her evaluate any recommendations.

6-1 In doing breast self-examination, women occasionally discover fibrous growths which feel like peeled grapes or bath oil beads. These harmless, fluid-filled pockets, called cysts, can be tiny, or as large as a walnut. The growth of cysts often seems to be related to the menstrual cycle and women who take hormone-like drugs (such as the Pill) are definitely more prone to them.

Breast cysts are not serious and, unless they hurt or grow very large, they can be left alone. Some cysts can grow and shrink during the menstrual cycle. Many women find it reassuring to learn to recognize cysts during a physical examination. From then on, they can monitor them on their own.

6-2 Genital warts (also called venereal warts) are caused by a virus and are like any other warts. They are sometimes transmitted by sexual contact and both heterosexual women and lesbians can get them. They have no feeling when touched, but can itch and bleed and can be pulled away from the skin when they are scratched. Vigorous sex or tight-fitting pants can irritate them.

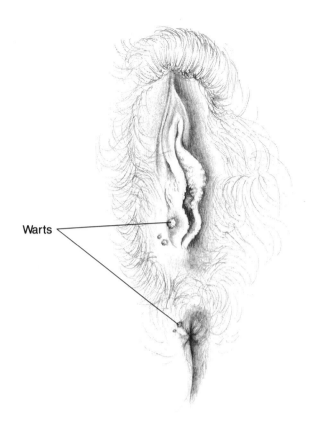

Warts

If not treated, the warts multiply in cauliflowerlike clusters and spread to other parts of the genitals. The usual treatment in either a clinic or doctor's office is podophyllum, a caustic resin which effectively kills the virus. A more drastic treatment burns off the warts.

6–3 Two lima-bean-sized glands on either side of the vaginal opening are the vulvovaginal or Bartholin's glands.

6–4 Occasionally, one or both become infected and can quickly swell to the size of a walnut. Like the appendix, the vulvovaginal glands don't seem to have any particular function and are only noticed when they cause trouble.

6–2   Genital warts

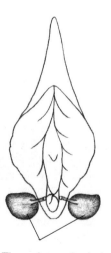

6–3   The vulvovaginal glands

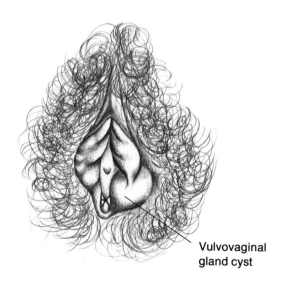

Vulvovaginal
gland cyst

6–4   A vulvovaginal gland cyst

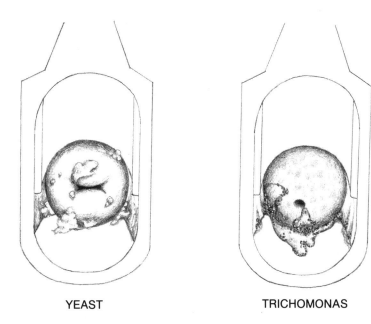

YEAST   TRICHOMONAS

6–5 Discharge from an overgrowth of yeast and from trichomonas

There are several home remedies which self-helpers have used to treat infected vulvovaginal glands. Sitz baths, or sitting in a tub with goldenseal-root powder, or applying a paste of goldenseal-root powder can help reduce the swelling and aid healing.

The usual medical remedy is to lance and drain the cyst and prescribe antibiotics to cure the infection.

6–5 Every woman has yeast in her vagina at all times. When it overgrows, it can cause burning on urination, itching and a heavy, clumpy discharge, sometimes described as "cottage-cheesy." Usually, medications do not work as well as a simple home remedy: yogurt. Unpasteurized, plain yogurt contains *Lactobacillus acidophilus*, a "friendly" bacteria which keeps the growth of yeast within a normal range. A common cause of a yeast condition is taking antibiotics, killing off all bacteria and allowing the yeast to multiply without competition. Replacing the *Lactobacillus* usually reduces the growth of yeast and the symptoms disappear.

The best way to insert yogurt is with a small spoon or spatula and a plastic speculum. The speculum also allows you to see how much yeasty secretion there is. Other methods of inserting yogurt are with the tip of a tampon, with your finger or in a vaginal-cream applicator. You can also make a douche from yogurt and water.

The secretion from a trichomonas infection is yellow or greenish in color and has a foul odor. In a severe infection, the cervix is covered with a heavy discharge. The most common home remedy for "trich" is a Betadine (povidone-iodine) douche, an antibacterial agent available at the drugstore. Other douches can be made from goldenseal or myrrh (one teaspoon to a quart of water), a chickweed bath (several handfuls in a tub) or you can make a garlic suppository. (A peeled garlic clove wrapped in gauze and inserted like a tampon. It's a good idea to leave a tail on the gauze like the string of a tampon, so that the suppository can be retrieved easily.)

Doctors use the catchall term "nonspecific vaginitis" to describe a variety of bacterial infections in the vagina. Some of the names you will hear for bacterial infections are *E. coli, Hemophilus, Gardnerella vaginalis,* strep and staph. Usually, a heavy discharge from an overgrowth of some type of bacteria will be yellowish to greenish and runny and have a strong odor.

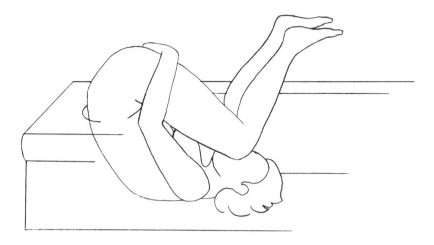

6–6 Sucking air: A technique to aid in the application of vaginal remedies

The home remedy that self-helpers often suggest is the same as for trichomonas. Other reliable remedies are the old standby, vinegar and water douche (one tablespoon of vinegar to one quart of warm water) and goldenseal or other herbal douches.

6–6 One highly effective technique a self-helper developed to aid in the application of vaginal remedies is called "sucking air." In the bathtub, she lies on her back at a 45-degree angle, with bent knees as close to her head as possible. She relaxes all of the muscles in her lower body, then applies a douche. This position allows the pelvic organs to fall away from the vagina and causes the vagina to balloon. Then the douche, which can be warmed to body temperature, is poured into the vagina where it must remain for several minutes until it overflows. This position allows the liquid to reach every nook and cranny of the vagina. If you have tried every other remedy and still have recurrences, you might want to try this.

6–7 Herpes is related to the virus which causes cold sores. It was thought that herpes occurred only in the genital area, but now it is clear that it can occur on other parts of the body as well. Some researchers now think that the herpes virus lives deep in the body in the nerve ganglia.

Herpes is most often contracted through sexual contact with someone who has active sores, but it can be picked up in other ways. It has reached epidemic proportions now, and there is no known cure. Once a person develops the sores, the virus remains in the body and can be activated at any time—when resistance is lowered or under stressful conditions.

Herpes, like pimples, is fairly easy to identify. Active sores can be seen around the mouth or genital area. Although the first bout is often the worst, any bout can be accompanied by miserable flulike symptoms that can last anywhere from one to six weeks. Active sores are a serious concern for a pregnant mother about to deliver, because the baby can pick up the virus as it passes down the birth canal.

There is no medication that will cure herpes, but there are a number of drugs and self-help remedies which can make the sores less painful and speed healing.

One of the newest and most promising home remedies which seems to both lessen the severity and promote healing of herpes is lysine, available in pill form at health food stores. Be careful to check ingredients: lysine is often found in combination with arginine, which seems to promote the growth of herpes.

Women who have herpes have found that certain vitamins such as B-complex, C, E and A help some-

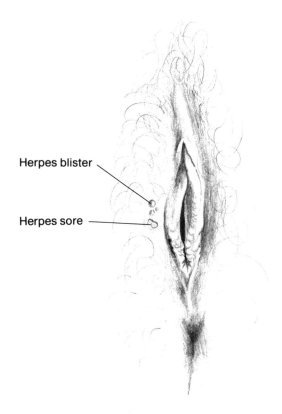

Herpes blister

Herpes sore

6–7 A group of active herpes blisters

what in preventing recurrences. They are particularly useful at time of stress. Women have noticed that a healthy diet and rest can be as important as anything in recovering from a major outbreak.

Some over-the-counter topical ointments can make the sores less painful. Neosporin ointment is an anesthetic and CamphoPhenique, zinc oxide and povidone-iodine (Betadine) can aid healing of sores.

Other herbal remedies, which self-helpers have found especially helpful in making the blisters less painful and which also aid in healing, are goldenseal, myrrh, comfrey root, aloe vera and peppermint tea.

Sitz baths can help keep the blisters clean, and drying them well afterward is very important.

Women who have had no luck with home remedies have resorted to prescription drugs, with varying success. Xylocaine jelly (an anesthetic), sulfa cream or Stoxil, usually prescribed for herpes in the eyes, can be used. Note: Stoxil is a very strong drug which has many physical effects and should not be used by pregnant women. Pyridium, a drug usually used for urinary tract infections, can help make urination less painful when a woman has active blisters. An experimental cream, called 2-deoxy *d*-glucose (2-DDG) has been found to inhibit the growth of active sores and

to shorten the duration of an outbreak.

Some remedies seem to work for some people and for others not at all. Frequent outbreaks of herpes can indicate an underlying health problem such as hypoglycemia, liver problems or adrenal exhaustion, that must be identified and treated before any progress can be made toward lessening the frequency of recurrences. Some people have found relief from constant attacks only after making radical changes in their diets or lifestyles. One prelude to establishing a new diet which some people have found beneficial is a liquid fast or detoxification diet and the elimination of sugar, white flour, stimulants and additives. Holistic practitioners and nutritionists can often be helpful in making major dietary changes.

Several people who suffer from severe monthly herpes attacks have reported that they were able to suppress the outbreaks only after going on long-term detoxification diets supervised by holistic nutritionists. Specific supplements they found helpful, in addition to vitamins, were lysine, lactobacillus acidophilus (fresh), fatty acids or vitamin F, calcium lactate, and a special homeopathic preparation for herpes treatment.

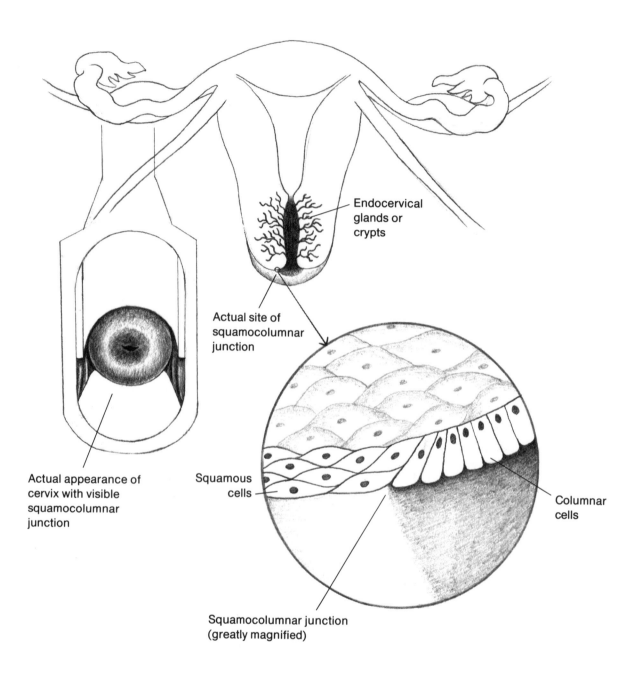

Endocervical
glands or
crypts

Actual site of
squamocolumnar
junction

Actual appearance of
cervix with visible
squamocolumnar
junction

Squamous
cells

Columnar
cells

Squamocolumnar junction
(greatly magnified)

6–8   The squamocolumnar junction

6-8 The place on the cervix where the long, col-umn-shaped cells of the cervical canal meet the flat cells of the face of the cervix is called the squamo-columnar junction. The cells of the canal are dark red and the cells of the surface are pink. The difference is as striking as that between the lip and facial skin. Sometimes this junction occurs on the face of the cer-vix, and the bright red circle of the cells of the canal can be mistaken for cervicitis or cervical erosion.

Often, physicians mistakenly want to remove the red cells, which can get darker or lighter during the men-strual cycle. The squamocolumnar junction, whether it occurs deep within the canal or on the face of the cervix, is the most common site of abnormal growth of cells which might eventually develop into cancer, so it is important for a woman to have regular Pap smears from this area.

6-9 Sometimes bacteria, from gonorrhea or other

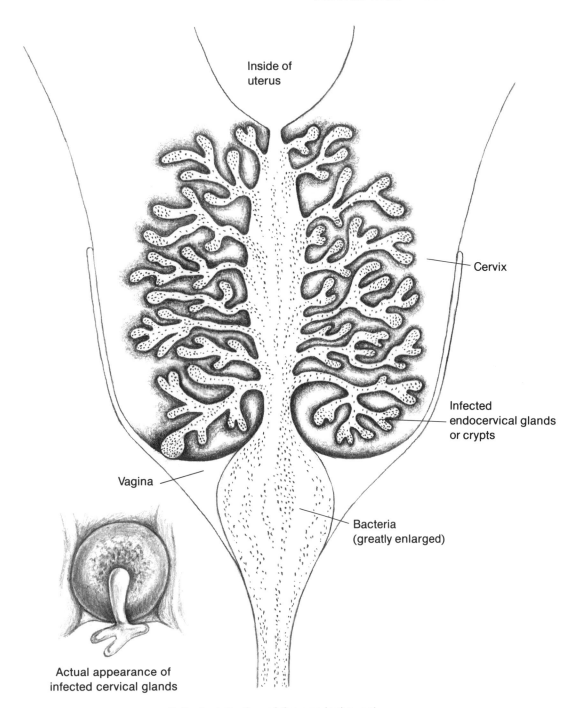

Inside of
uterus

Cervix

Infected
endocervical glands
or crypts

Vagina

Bacteria
(greatly enlarged)

Actual appearance of
infected cervical glands

6–9   An infection of the cervical canal

bacterial inflammation, can enter the cervical canal. This will cause the cervix to become red and tender and will produce a very heavy discharge. Even though the general infection may be cleared up, some bacteria can hide in the tiny crypts and crevices of the canal and flare up again. A lot of women use a diaphragm or cervical cap to hold home remedy medications against the cervix to promote healing. Betadine, goldenseal, vitamin E oil and honey are useful as well as soothing. Some severe cervical infections are caused by chlamydia, a virus-like bacteria which is difficult to identify unless a laboratory has the ability to culture viruses. Chlamydia lives in the cervical cells and is not responsive to home remedies. Women who are on the Pill have a higher incidence of this type of infecton, which has also been identified as a cause of urinary tract infections and pelvic inflammatory disease.

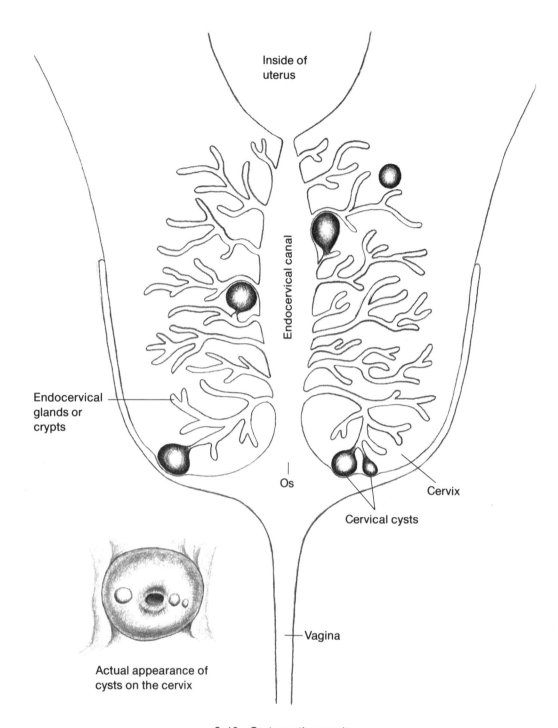

6–10   Cysts on the cervix

6–10 Cysts are common in many parts of the body and they can also appear in the endocervical canal where they are not visible, even with a speculum. No one knows what causes cysts, but one theory is that they are the body's way of containing infection. In the cervical canal or on the face of the cervix, they can be the size of a pinhead or the size of a pea, and can grow and shrink throughout the menstrual cycle. Generally, these cysts do not hurt and do not cause serious problems, so most women just leave them alone.

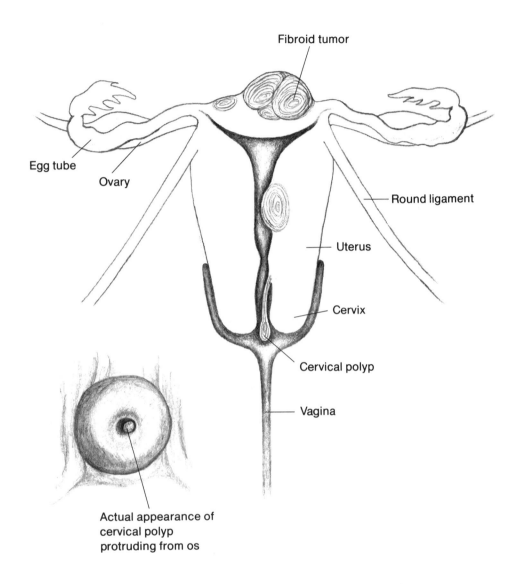

Fibroid tumor

Egg tube

Ovary

Round ligament

Uterus

Cervix

Cervical polyp

Vagina

Actual appearance of
cervical polyp
protruding from os

6–11   Uterine fibroids and cervical polyps

6-11 Fibroid tumors are dense fibrous growths which develop within or on the surface of the uterus. In doing a uterine size check a health worker, nurse or doctor can feel hard lumps on the smooth outer surface of the uterus. Polyps are similar to fibroids but have stems and do not grow so large. They often grow in the cervical canal and can sometimes be seen sticking out of the opening, and may bleed. If they change or grow, they can be removed by a physician.

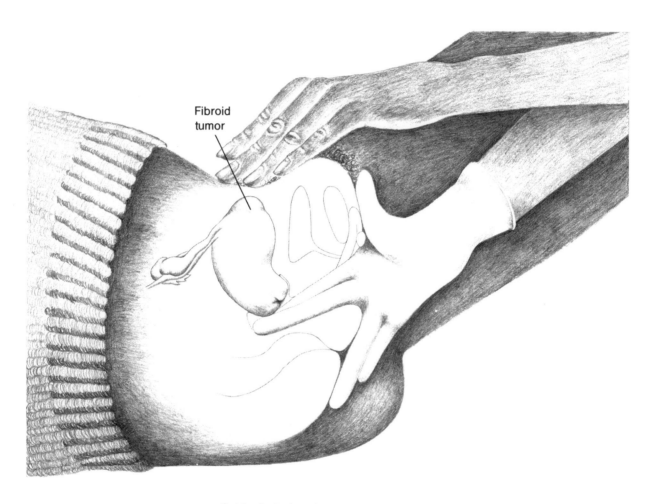

Fibroid
tumor

6–12 A uterine size check for fibroids

6-12 Most women never know that they have fibroids until they are discovered by a physician during a uterine size check. They don't hurt and they aren't dangerous, but if they grow large, they can cause pain. Fibroids can press on nerves or on the bladder or colon and interfere with the proper functioning of these organs. Sometimes they can cause heavy uterine bleeding and discharge and they can also cause miscarriage. Physicians generally recommend removal of the fibroids by a procedure called myomectomy if you are not pregnant, and they almost always insist on a cesarean delivery if you are and want to continue your pregnancy.

No one knows positively what causes menstrual cramps, possibly because researchers have not been particularly interested in doing research on the menstrual cycle. No one knows why some women do not have any cramps at all or why some have very painful menstruation, which doctors call dysmenorrhea. Self-helpers have observed that cramps seem to come from the uterus's powerful muscular contractions which force blood, uterine lining and clots through the tiny bottleneck of the cervical canal.

Recent research suggests that women who have severe cramps have higher levels of substances called prostaglandins, which stimulate uterine contractions. Some physicians have had limited success in prescribing a drug called Ponstel which prevents the manufacture of prostaglandins, but so far, research is too scanty to draw any conclusions. Women who have very severe cramps are often willing to try any new remedy, but we are wary of doctors prescribing new "wonder drugs" without sufficient research on the possible ill effects.

Doctors often diagnose painful periods as endometriosis, a condition in which bits of tissue from the uterine lining grow outside the uterus in other parts of the pelvic cavity. This diagnosis is a guess, since it would take extensive surgery to locate such tissue.

In addition to menstrual pain and muscle spasms, other typical menstrual symptoms are bloating from water retention, headache, depression and constipation. Physicians routinely prescribe diuretics for fluid retention, pain killers and tranquilizers, and even stimulants. Some physicians have even experimented with prescribing estrogen-like drugs as an antidote for severe menstrual symptoms or for endometriosis. The major effect of this prescription is to make ovulation stop, thus stopping menstruation and menstrual cramps, replacing them with monthly withdrawal bleeding.

There are a number of home remedies which many women have used to lessen the discomfort of severe cramps and other menstrual symptoms. Some women have found that completely avoiding salt, and drinking herbal teas, (particularly yarrow), eating lightly and doing strenuous exercise lessen the severity of cramps. Women who do regular, strenuous exercise find that their cramps gradually lessen and their periods become lighter. There is also a series of simple exercises which can relax muscles and readjust internal organs. Some women have found that an orgasm helps to get rid of heavy cramps.

6-13 One technique to reduce muscle tension is to consciously relax muscle groups from toe to scalp in succession. Lie on a firm surface, rest your head on one pillow and elevate your legs over another. To relax, concentrate on letting each succeeding set of muscles become limp and loose. Relaxing the outer muscles can help relax the uterus, which is also a muscle.

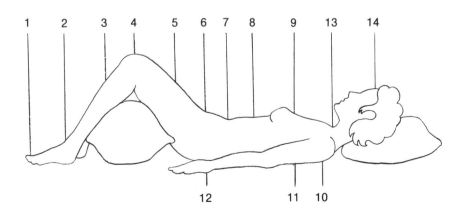

6-13 A relaxation technique to relieve menstrual cramps

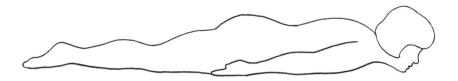

6–14 First step of the cobra exercise to relieve menstrual cramps

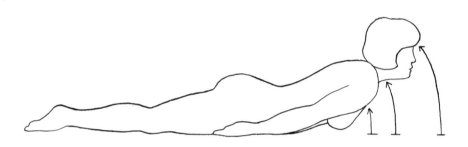

6–15 Second step of the cobra exercise

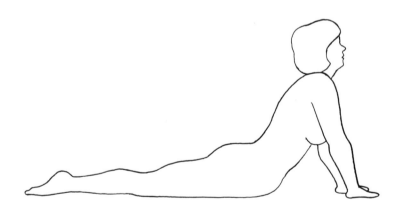

6–16 Third step of the cobra exercise

6-14 The cobra exercise can be used to help relieve lower back pain. The first step is to lie flat on a hard surface such as the floor.

6-15 Gradually raise your head and chest without using your arms until your torso is off the floor.

6-16 Now use your arms to raise your torso so that your back is arched. Repeat this several times until the lower back muscles relax.

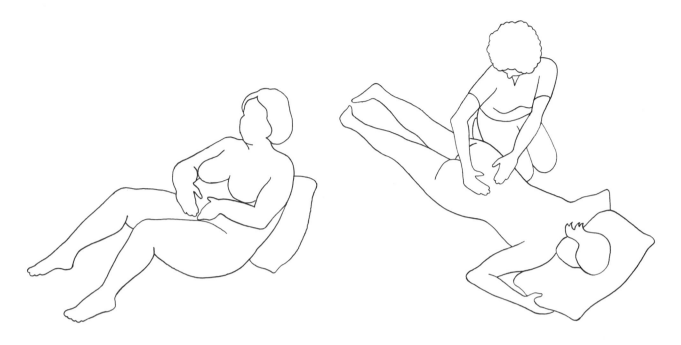

6-17 Direct uterine massage to relieve menstrual cramps

6-18 Lower back massage to relieve menstrual cramps

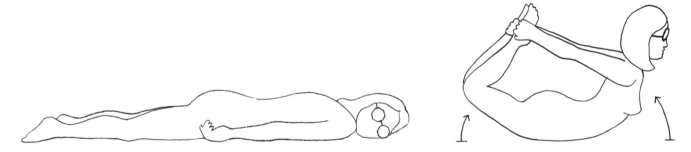

6-19 First step of the bow exercise to relieve menstrual cramps

6-20 Second step of the bow exercise

6-17 Another technique that helps the uterus relax is direct uterine massage. You can do this yourself, or with the help of a friend or partner. Press on the spot just above the pubic hairline where the uterus is and massage gently. Women have noticed that this often helps the uterus push out a large clot and thus relieve cramps.

6-18 Having someone apply pressure directly to the lower back often helps relieve the tension caused by pressure on nerves and the spinal column.

6-19 The bow is a yoga exercise that is also helpful for releasing muscle tension. Begin by lying flat on a firm surface.

6-20 Grasp your ankles with both hands and pull them toward the back of your head. Gently rock back and forth, stretching tense muscles. Repeat several times until tension goes away.

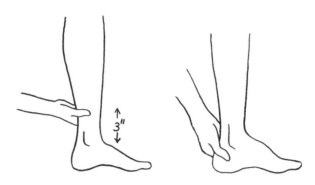

6-21 Direct pressure point massage to relieve menstrual cramps

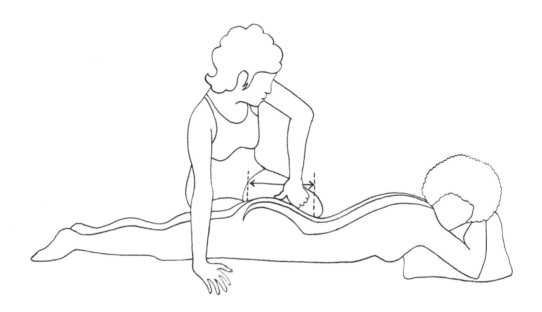

6-22 *Shiatsu* massage to relieve menstrual cramps

6-21 Direct pressure applied to the Achilles tendon often seems to help lessen tension and discomfort in the pelvic area. With the thumb and forefinger about three inches above the heel, press firmly for ten to 15 seconds. Release and press again on the other ankle.

6-22 *Shiatsu,* another form of pressure point massage, can also be used. It requires that another person press, with the flat of the thumb, on the side of each vertebra from the end of the spine to the waist. Increase the pressure gradually and, after about ten seconds, decrease it slowly.

6-23 A urinary tract infection (UTI), or cystitis, is one of the most bothersome conditions a woman can have. Frequency of urination, burning upon urination and blood in the urine are the usual symptoms, and they can be accompanied by fever, chills and fatigue.

The causes of UTI can be sexual activity, trauma to the urethra, bacterial infections in the vagina or stress. Recent research has shown that chlamydia, a virus-like bacteria, is a frequent cause of UTI. The illustration here shows the kidneys, which are near the small

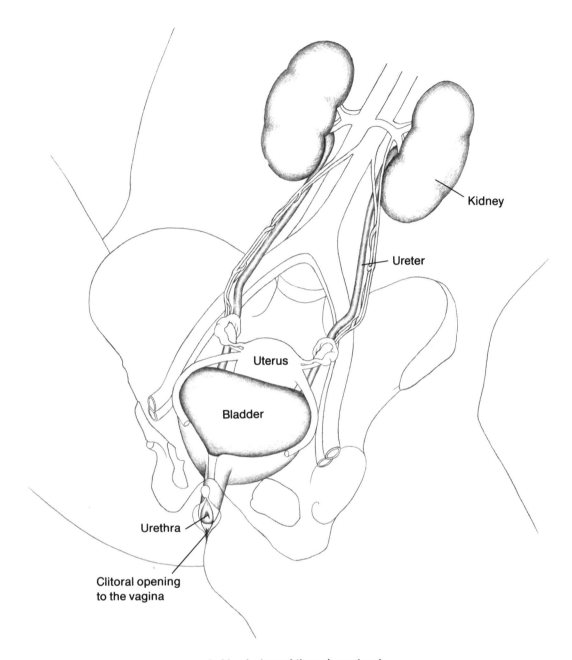

Kidney

Ureter

Uterus

Bladder

Urethra

Clitoral opening
to the vagina

6–23 A view of the urinary tract

of the back, and a full bladder in front of the uterus and slightly lower.

The standard home remedy for bladder infections is to drink large quantities of water or cranberry juice, preferably without sugar, for two or three days. This flushes the bladder of the irritating bacteria that are causing spasms and burning. All acidic liquids, tea, coffee, soft drinks, citrus juice and alcohol should be avoided completely, since they make the bladder a more hospitable place for bacteria to live. If the symptoms reappear, especially if blood is present, it is usually necessary to take antibacterial agents in order to get rid of the infection quickly and completely. One unfortunate side effect of taking antibacterial agents, especially antibiotics, can be a yeast condition.

Some women are plagued by UTI for years and can lessen its frequency only by identifying the source of chronic irritation.

6-24 In the fall of 1980, it was reported that a number of women had been stricken by a mysterious disease called toxic shock syndrome (TSS) and that 40 women had died from it. The Center for Disease Control (CDC) suspects that the cause of this rare but deadly condition is staph bacteria, possibly a new strain of the *Staphylococcus aureus* family to which the body may not be resistant. Nearly all women who were stricken with TSS were using tampons and a large proportion had used Rely or other super-absorbent varieties, including Playtex and Tampax. A few men and children have also been found to have TSS. The most common symptoms of toxic shock syndrome are diarrhea, vomiting, high fever, a drop in blood pressure and a sunburnlike rash.

This illustration shows five different kinds of tampons: Rely (expanded), OB, Kotex, Tampax and Playtex (from left to right). Rely was withdrawn from the market after it was implicated in TSS reactions. Many women will, of course, continue to use the tampons which are available. If you do choose to use them, CDC recommends frequently alternating them with napkins. They also recommend not using the super-absorbent type. Or you may want to try an alternative method of catching the menstrual flow.

Below, left, is a menstrual sponge. The Women's Health Movement has revived the use of sea sponges to absorb the menstrual flow. Although one woman who developed TSS was using a menstrual sponge, we still feel that it is a viable alternative to tampons. Certainly it is cheaper and longer lasting. The sponge can be trimmed to a comfortable size and inserted by pushing it into the vagina with a finger. It can be removed after several hours, rinsed and reinserted immediately. If you have difficulty in removing it, as some women do, you can run a thread or a bit of dental floss through one end to use like a tampon string. If the sponge develops an odor, it can be soaked for a few minutes in vinegar and water or baking soda and water. Some women have found that the diaphragm is also a useful way to catch the flow. Like a sponge, it can be rinsed and used again immediately.

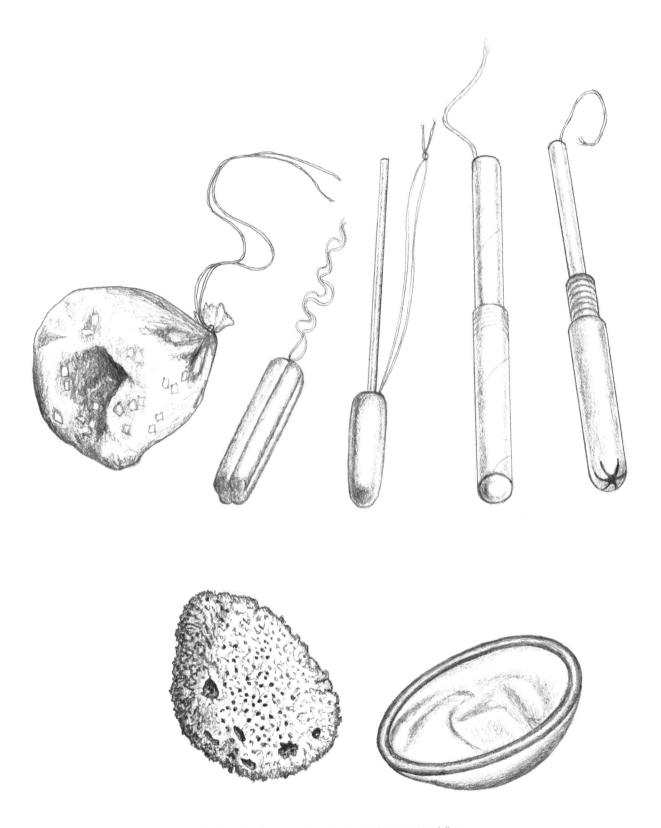

6–24   Devices to absorb or catch menstrual flow

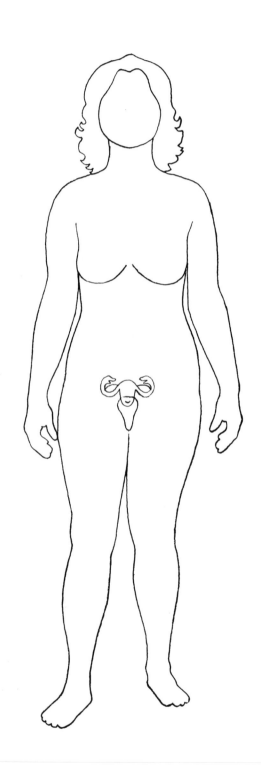

7 • Birth Control

The choice of birth control is a complicated one and, unfortunately, a decision is often made because the doctor or clinic happens to prefer a certain method. It is no accident that some doctors are known as "Pill doctors" or as "IUD doctors." On the other hand, women's clinics are well known for encouraging women to try local and natural methods of birth control and for emphasizing the diaphragm and cervical cap. The problem of birth control is a difficult one: in addition to the limitation of choices, what is suitable at one period of a woman's life may not be suitable at other times.

Many women find that any method of birth control becomes more effective when they have information about their reproductive organs and about the method they have chosen. Myths about various methods simply evaporate when women look into their vaginas for the first time. One myth, for example, is that of a lost diaphragm.

The object of all methods, of course, is to prevent the sperm and egg from uniting or from implanting on the uterine wall. No method today, except hysterectomy, can totally ensure this outcome.

After ovulation, the egg makes its journey about halfway down the egg tube where it stops for three to four days. It then moves to the lower third of the tube, where it stays for one or two days and where the egg and sperm usually meet. After the man ejaculates, some sperm will find their way into the cervical glands and will be released over the next three to five days. If there is fertile mucus, sperm can live for as many as five days in the cervical canal where they are released gradually to travel through the uterus to the egg tubes. Thus, a pregnancy can result from coitus around the time of ovulation or even before, although fertilization does not occur until five to six days later. This newly discovered ability of cervical mucus to nurture and transport sperm is one factor in explaining the 20-percent failure rate of the rhythm method. There is also *no* guarantee that a woman will ovulate only once in a cycle. Likewise, it is thought that women do not ovulate every single cycle of their reproductive years. In short, ovulation is not a cut-and-dried event for every woman, all the time.

The trouble with the most widely distributed methods of birth control—the Pill and the IUD—is that they both have severe and long-lasting physical effects for some women, and neither is any more effective than less harmful methods.

The Pill works by chemically causing a state in which the activity of the ovaries is suppressed so that a woman does not ovulate. For many women, this condition lasts from three to six months after they stop taking the Pill and *can* last up to a year and a half or longer. A few women's ovaries never ovulate or produce normal levels of hormones again.

When the Pill was first marketed, women did not bleed at all, and they didn't like it. So drug manufacturers "doctored" the Pill so women would have cyclic bleeding. This blood, however, is not a period. It is drug-withdrawal bleeding promoted by abruptly discontinuing the hormone-like drugs, either by not taking Pills for seven days or by taking sugar pills.

No one knows exactly *how* the IUD works. It may actually scrape the implantation off of the uterine wall; or it may cause a low-grade infection in the uterus, creating numerous white blood cells which may kill the sperm; or it may cause the uterus to contract continuously in an effort to expel the foreign object within, and thus expel any implantation as well. Some women have found that taking aspirin or antibiotics renders their IUDs temporarily ineffective.

The incidence of serious infection with the IUD is a concern for many women. Pelvic infections strike fast and are difficult to cure and can cause scarring of the tubes and ovaries. Once a woman has had a severe pelvic infection, she is more prone to recurrence.

It is generally recommended that a woman have her IUD changed every three years. This routine replacement seems to have originated with the widespread use of the Copper-7 IUD, which supposedly needs to be replaced when all of the copper has been absorbed by the body. The exact role that copper plays in preventing pregnancy is unknown. Very occasionally, women who have had their IUDs for more than three years experience difficulty in removal, because some tissue has begun to grow around the body of the IUD. The copper itself may be intrinsically dangerous, and no one knows the long-term effects of a continual release of copper in the body. However, if you are not having any trouble with your current IUD and do not wish to experience the discomfort of removal and insertion, you may choose to keep the one you have as long as the string is visible.

Sometimes, women who have never had children have more severe cramps or pain with their IUDs and have to have them removed, although women who have had children also have this experience. It is possible that even the smallest IUD is not small enough for some women. It is impossible to predict in advance which women will be able to tolerate an IUD and which will not.

Because of the dangers of the Pill and IUD, barrier and natural methods of birth control are becoming more popular. Barrier methods—the diaphragm, condoms and the cervical cap—work well because they present a physical shield between the penis and the cervix.

The choice of a birth control method is a significant decision for any woman and it must often be made on the basis of incomplete information about various methods and with little information about our reproductive cycles. The factors involved in choosing a method are numerous: Will it prevent pregnancy? Does it have harmful physical effects? Is it convenient? Will my partner or partners complain? Does it require partner cooperation? Can I get stranded without it? How expensive is it? Will it affect my ability to have children in the future? How much time and effort does it require? If this method doesn't work or I don't like it or my partner doesn't like it, what will I choose then?

Some women find that one method which works quite well during one period of their lives is completely inappropriate if their circumstances change. Even though a woman has made a decision, it often needs to be reevaluated to take into account both changing circumstances and the success she has had with her chosen method.

Knowing about fertile mucus is of more value than mere theoretical interest. Knowledge of the specific time when you are fertile can be vitally important—if you want to avoid pregnancy or if you want to become pregnant.

The "mucus observation," "fertility detection" or "fertility awareness" method of birth control depends upon watching for the time in the cycle when fertile mucus is present. The symptothermic method combines mucus observation with the basal body temperature method (charting the temperature every morning upon waking). For many women, this double observation, of fertile mucus and of temperature pattern, gives a reasonably good indication of when their fertile times occur. If the stretchy fertile mucus is present at the same time that temperature makes a sharp rise and then a drop, then there is a very high probability that ovulation has occurred.

You may find this method difficult because your temperature does not show a clear pattern. In this case, observations over a period of several months are necessary to see if the pattern is reliable.

Individual women or couples who are willing to devote more time to the subject of birth control have had success with natural methods such as mucus or cycle observation, basal body temperature or the rhythm or calendar method, and even some unconventional methods like lunaception and astrological computation.

Different methods of birth control affect different parts of the body. It is important for women to know exactly what those effects are and how long they last.

7-1 The basal body temperature method is a natural method in which you take your temperature upon waking each morning, using a chart and a special thermometer which is easy to read and available at

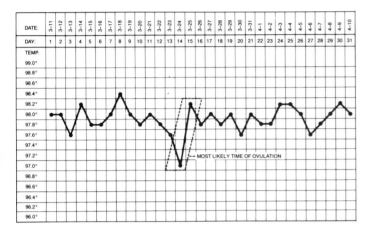

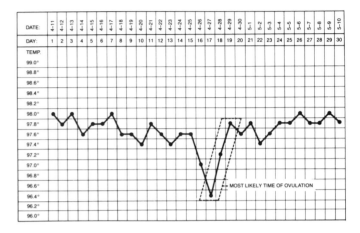

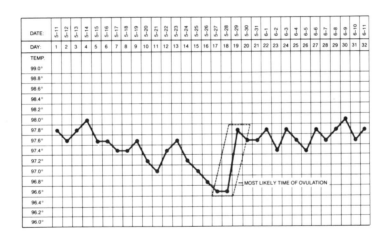

7–1   A basal body temperature chart

any drugstore. Prior to ovulation, your temperature drops, then rises, either sharply or gradually, at the time of ovulation. The difference between the lower and higher temperatures is about 0.3 to 0.6 degree. However, some women have reported a difference of one degree or more. After three days of the higher temperature, it is assumed that ovulation has occurred. Then the higher temperature will drop slightly just before menstruation begins. After taking your temperature for several months, you can often see a pattern develop. If you find that you ovulate regularly, then you can use a local method of birth control or keep the penis out of the vagina until you think your fertile time is over. Many women have had excellent results by combining the basal body temperature method with mucus observation. Although it requires more effort and time than some other methods, many women or couples who do not want to assume certain health risks along with birth control have found it quite satisfactory.

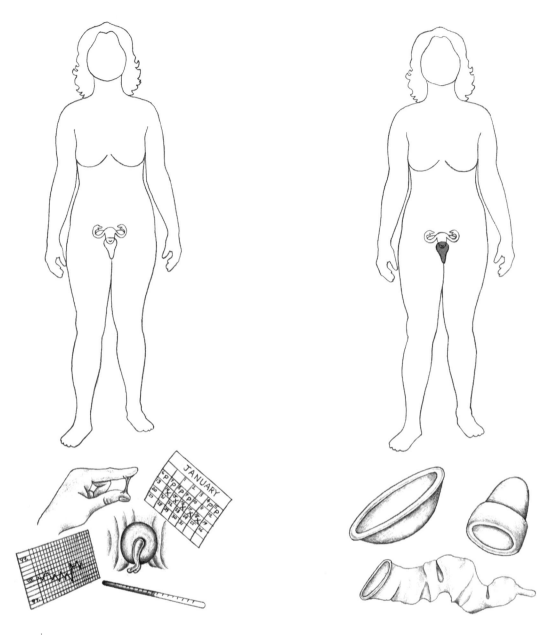

7–2   The effects of self-observation as birth control

7–3   The effects of local methods as birth control

7-2 Natural methods which emphasize self-obser-vation or abstinence do not have any undesirable physical effects.

7-3 The effects of local methods, which include the diaphragm, cervical cap and condom, are confined to the vagina. The vagina is a mucous membrane which absorbs a bit of the substances with which it comes into contact. If you use a garlic suppository, for exam-ple, you will be able to taste garlic in your mouth. So far there is not very much evidence to suggest that the

use of spermicides in the vagina is harmful in any way. In fact, preliminary findings suggest that the di-aphragm actually protects against precancerous cervi-cal conditions.

7-4 IUDs are placed in the uterus, and they can have harmful and even severe effects. Women who use IUDs tend to have more vaginal infections and a dramatically higher rate of uterine infections, which can spread quickly to the tubes and ovaries and are difficult to cure. Occasionally, an infection also affects

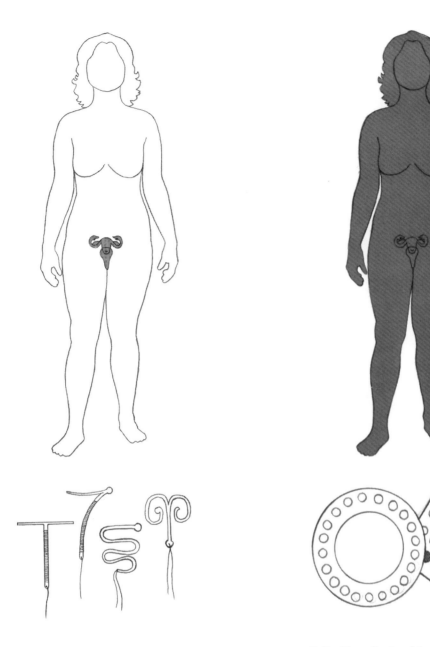

7–4   The effects of IUDs as birth control

7–5   The effects of the pill as birth control

the entire abdominal cavity. Sometimes the infection is so severe that the only cure is a hysterectomy. Although a large number of women who begin using the IUD stop within the first year, some are able to use it successfully for several years.

7-5 The visible undesirable effects of the Pill are minimal for many women. Fluid retention, weight gain, headaches and mood changes are regarded as nuisances. For other women, the effects are severe, including blood clots, strokes, severe headaches and depression. In the long range, women who take the Pill have a significantly higher incidence of several types of cancer, including cancer of the breast, uterus and cervix. When taking the Pill, danger signs are: changes in vision, chest pains, shortness of breath, severe leg cramps, chest or arm pain, jaundice (yellow color of the skin or whites of the eyes), severe depression with no other explanation and a sensation of flashing lights.

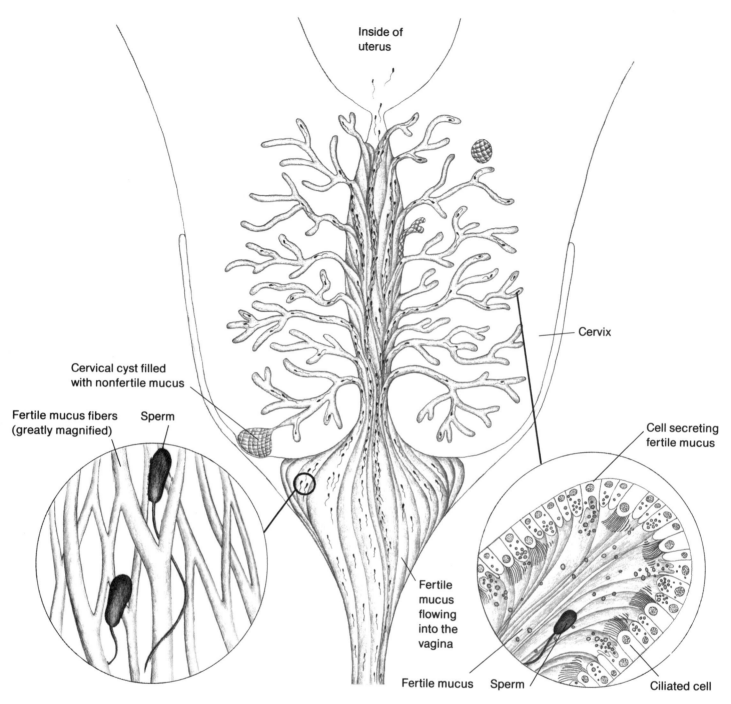

Inside of uterus

Cervical cyst filled
with nonfertile mucus

Fertile mucus fibers
(greatly magnified)   Sperm

Cervix

Cell secreting
fertile mucus

Fertile
mucus
flowing
into the
vagina

Fertile mucus   Sperm

Ciliated cell

7–6A   Inset: The structure
of fertile mucus

7–6   A cross section of the cervix with fertile mucus

7–6B   Inset: An endocervical
gland with fertile mucus

7-6, 7-6A, 7-6B Fertile mucus is a special type of mucus present around the time of ovulation. This cross section of the cervix shows the makeup of fertile mucus and of sperm passing through the cervical canal into the uterus. Fertile mucus is more alkaline than nonfertile mucus and better for sperm to survive in. It has parallel streams which suck the sperm up into the canal and into its myriad passages and crypts. Its consistency is stretchy, somewhat like egg white.

Women find it easiest to identify the difference by using a speculum. Fertile mucus usually appears as a clear bubble in the cervical os and will make a string of an inch or more between two points. For example, you can touch a cotton-tipped swab to the os and pull it back slowly or you can stretch the mucus between your fingers. Sperm can live in fertile mucus for up to five days and can thus arrive in the egg tube several days after a woman has coitus.

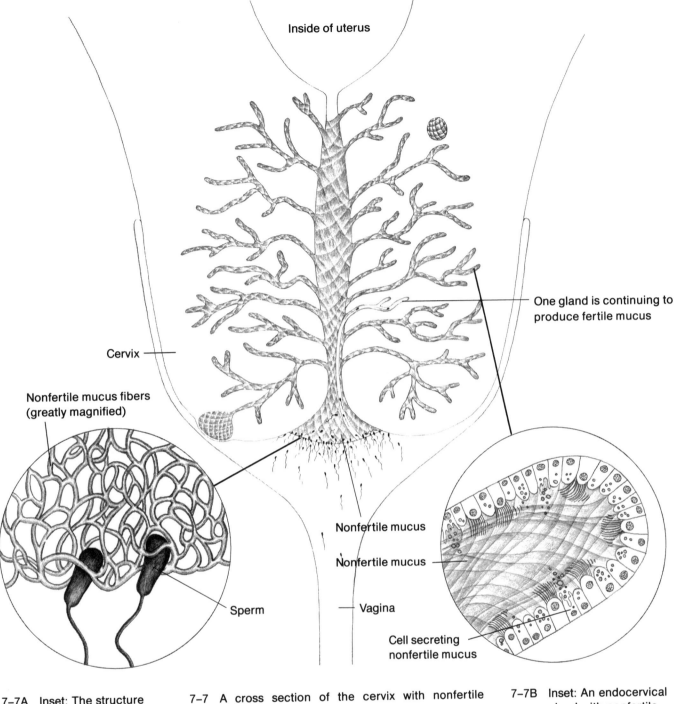

Inside of uterus

One gland is continuing to produce fertile mucus

Cervix

Nonfertile mucus fibers (greatly magnified)

Sperm

Nonfertile mucus

Nonfertile mucus

Vagina

Cell secreting nonfertile mucus

7–7A Inset: The structure of nonfertile mucus

7–7 A cross section of the cervix with nonfertile mucus

7–7B Inset: An endocervical gland with nonfertile mucus

Inset 7–6A shows the approximate structure of fertile mucus. It is composed of long, parallel passages which aid the sperm in their journey. Sometimes, women are very surprised to find fertile mucus at times other than the midpoint of their cycles. If it is present, it is safest to assume that another ovulation has occurred.

Inset 7–6B of an endocervical gland shows fertile mucus being produced. These glands are lined with column-shaped cells which burst, emptying mucus into the pool within. Some cells have hairlike projections, called cilia, which wave back and forth, pushing the mucus out of the passageways into the cervical canal.

7–7, 7–7A, 7–7B This cross section shows nonfertile mucus which is present in the cervical canal except when a woman ovulates. Some women find the changes in their mucus secretions very noticeable

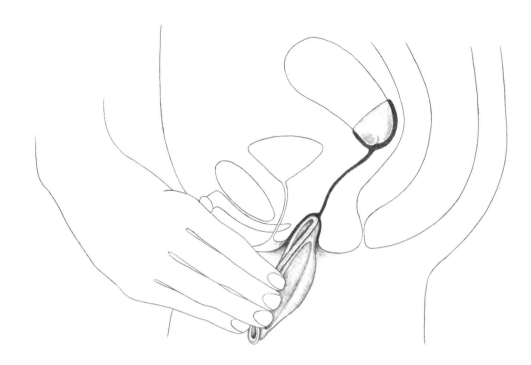

7–8   How to insert a diaphragm

around the time of ovulation, while others have difficulty in distinguishing any difference at all.

Inset 7–7A shows the crisscrossing woven structure of nonfertile mucus, which works as a barrier to sperm. When this type of mucus is present, only a few sperm are able to get into the cervical canal. Its acidic property also acts to kill the sperm.

Inset 7–7B shows an endocervical gland, greatly magnified, where nonfertile mucus is being manufactured.

7–8 Once you have done self-examination, you can easily see how a diaphragm works. The back rim of the diaphragm fits over the cervix and the front fits snugly behind the pubic bone just inside the vaginal opening. The rubber dome holds sperm-killing jelly or cream against the cervix. The diaphragm and other barrier methods are highly effective types of birth control, and have the added advantage of protection against infections and gonorrhea.

Some women or their partners feel that use of the diaphragm interferes with spontaneity because it must be inserted prior to coitus. It is possible to insert the diaphragm up to six hours before coitus is anticipated. Some women find that having more than one diaphragm, at least an extra one to carry in the purse or glove compartment of the car, helps to ensure that they will not be without birth control in unexpected circumstances. Some cream or jelly has a medicinal odor and taste, which some women or their partners object to. Although there aren't very many choices on the market, it does help to change brands until you find the most suitable one available.

7–9 You can check your diaphragm and thus make it more effective by inserting two fingers to feel if your cervix is covered by the rubber dome. One of the major reasons for diaphragm failure is that doctors often do not give women enough information for its most effective use. It is not uncommon for doctors to fail to show you how to check to see if your cervix is covered.

7–10 The diaphragm is usually removed by hooking the middle finger under the rim near the pubic bone and dislodging it, then pulling it out through the vaginal opening. Some women are not able to get it out this way, however, and have to invent their own ways, squatting down or perhaps sitting on a toilet.

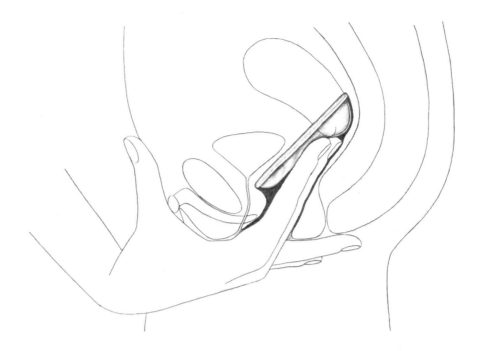

7-9   How to check a diaphragm

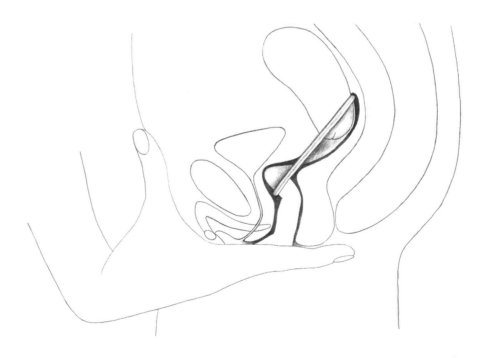

7-10   How to remove a diaphragm

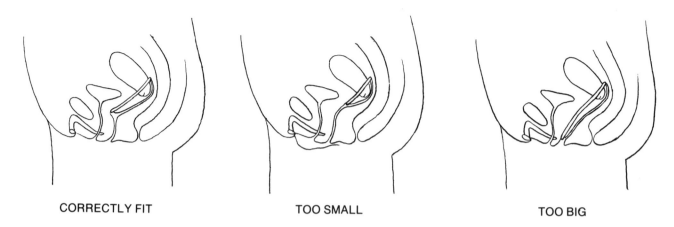

CORRECTLY FIT   TOO SMALL   TOO BIG

7-11   Correctly and incorrectly fit diaphragms

7-11 The diaphragm should cover the cervix and fit securely behind the pubic bone. If it is too small, it will move around in the vagina. If it is too large, it can be felt pressing against the vaginal walls.

In most women-controlled clinics, you actually fit yourself for a diaphragm, learn how to check to see if your cervix is covered, and thus leave with some experience in inserting and removing it.

7-12 Cervical caps have been a standard form of birth control in England for most of this century, and they enjoyed a brief but forgotten reign in this country before the advent of the Pill. They have been introduced again in the United States by a number of women-controlled clinics (see Appendix) and, increasingly, by a few doctors and nurse practitioners.

The cervical cap, which is held on the cervix by

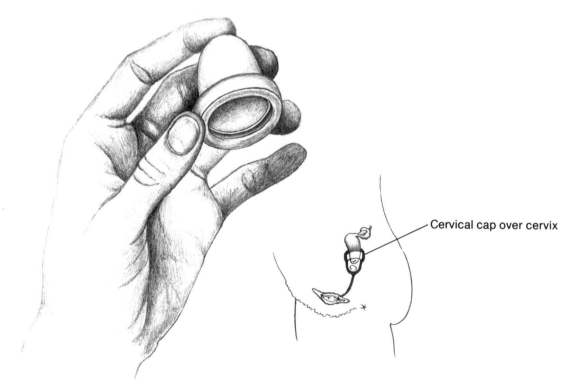

Cervical cap over cervix

7-12   The cervical cap

suction, comes in four sizes and is made of soft rubber. It requires only a little sperm-killing cream or jelly in the bottom third of the cap and can be left on for two or three days at a time. Like the diaphragm, the cap should remain in place for six to eight hours after coitus. Women's clinics believe that the cap is probably at least as effective as the diaphragm. The major negative aspect of the cap for some women is that it is difficult to remove. The suction can be broken by dislodging the cap from its place, or "burping" it like a plastic refrigerator container. Women with very short fingers or very long vaginas have had to invent ways to remove it. Some have found that a standard diaphragm applicator works perfectly. It can be used as an extension of the finger or by itself to help break the suction. You can run a loop of dental floss or heavy string through the little tab beneath the rim with a darning needle.

Another apparent drawback of the cap is that it only comes in four sizes and some women find it difficult to get a good fit. A large majority of women, however, wear one of the two medium sizes.

After use, the cap can be rinsed with soap and water and reinserted at that time or put away until needed again. If, as some women have noticed, an unpleasant odor develops, the cap can be soaked for 20 minutes or so in a cup of water with a tablespoon of baking soda, vinegar or lemon juice and then rinsed with water. Some women have found that a drop of chlorophyll inside the cap is a good preventive against odor.

7-13 The condom, like the diaphragm and cap, is a barrier method of birth control. It is made of soft rubber, sheep membrane or latex, fits snugly over a man's penis and has space at the end to catch the semen.

Sometimes semen can be spilled into the vagina if the man's penis becomes soft, but this can be avoided by holding the open end of the condom tightly around the penis as it is withdrawn and also by not withdrawing too long after ejaculation. If the condom does not have a reservoir at the end to catch the semen, it is good to leave a little space so that the semen will have some place to go.

Condoms used alone are about 90 percent effective in preventing pregnancy, but combined with foam or other spermicides, they are 99 percent effective. Except for an occasional allergic reaction to rubber, condoms do not have any undesirable physical effects and they actually help in preventing sexually transmitted diseases. A further advantage is that they are available in almost all drugstores or can be ordered by mail.

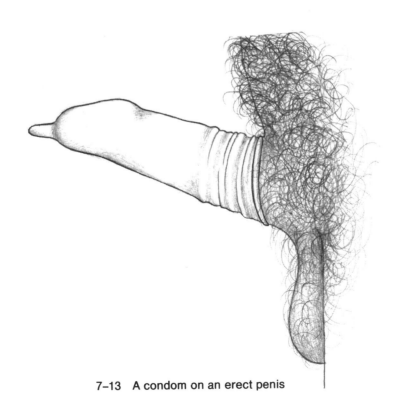

7-13   A condom on an erect penis

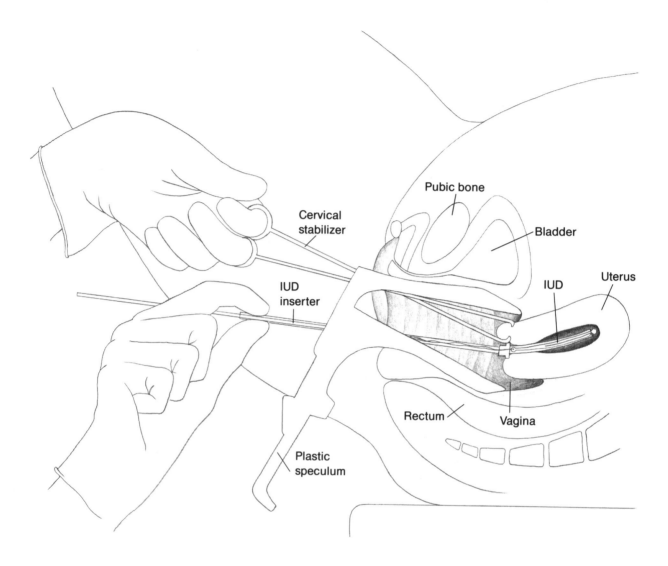

7-14 Step one of IUD insertion

7-14 IUDs are made of flexible plastic and have a string that hangs out of the os into the vagina so their presence can be checked. Some are wrapped with copper wire. The newer plastic IUDs also have barium in them which makes them visible on X-rays. The IUD can be inserted by either a doctor or a nurse practitioner in just a few minutes in a clinic or doctor's office. The IUD comes in its own sterile package, ready for insertion. A very thin, strawlike instrument with a plunger is used to straighten the IUD before it is inserted into the uterus.

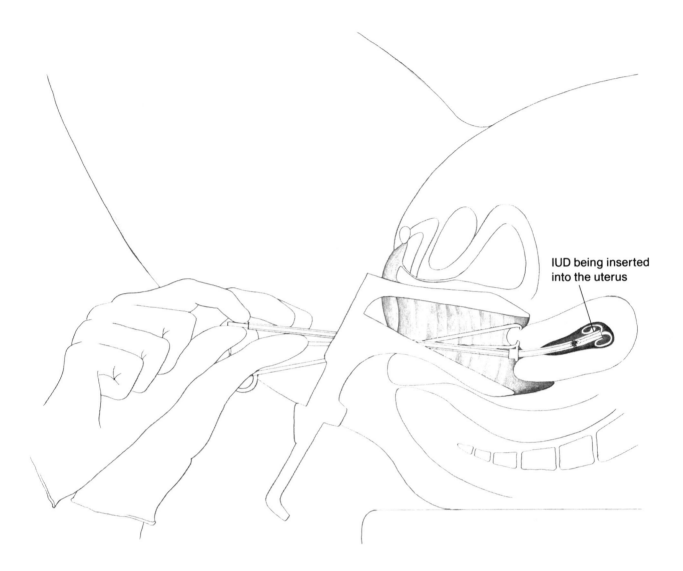

IUD being inserted
into the uterus

7–15 Step two of IUD insertion

7-15 The technician then pushes the plunger and the IUD emerges in the uterus and resumes its normal shape. One persistent myth about the IUD is that it must be inserted during your period. Physicians usually insist on this because the insertion can cause both cramping and bleeding. The os is a little more open during a woman's period, but it doesn't seem to make any substantial difference in how much cramping a woman feels. Some physicians also seem to think that you will notice cramping and bleeding less if you already have some.

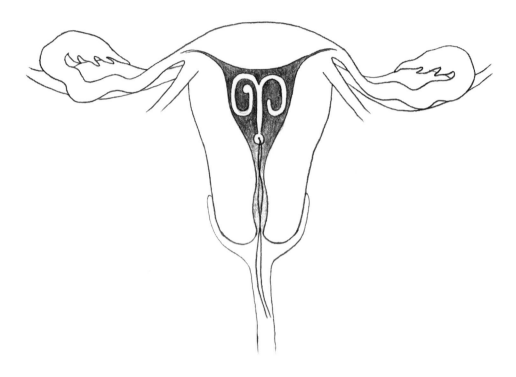

7–16   An IUD inserted

7–16 This picture shows a Saf-T-Coil IUD in place. There are five or six different kinds—and some experimental IUDs—and they come in various sizes. There doesn't seem to be any real difference among them, other than the possible ill effects of copper, as far as either comfort or effectiveness goes, so the choice between a Lippe's Loop, a Copper-7 or a Saf-T-Coil isn't really a major decision.

Many physicians show women how to check for their IUD string with a finger and recommend that they return within one to three months to have it checked, then every six months to a year after that. If you have a plastic speculum, you can check for yourself visually and know not only that it is there, but if it is still the same length, and you can see if there appears to be an infection developing.

Although the Dalkon Shield was removed from the U.S. market over ten years ago, its manufacturer did not recommend that all women who still had these IUDs in their uteruses have them removed until September, 1980, after more than 4,000 lawsuits had been filed against them.

BIRTH CONTROL

Method	*Description*	*% Effectiveness*
Abstinence	Keeping the penis out of the vagina. (Different from celibacy, which means not having sex with another person.)	100
Hysterectomy	Surgical removal of the uterus.	100
Vasectomy	Cutting or tying the tube which carries the sperm out of a man's penis.	99.85
Tubal Ligation	Cutting or burning the egg tubes or closing them off with a plastic ring.	99.4
Foam and Condom	The man fits a condom over his penis and the woman puts sperm-killing foam in her vagina.	99+*
Basal Body Temperature	Predicting a woman's fertile time by charting her early-morning temperature.	98.1
Diaphragm	A dome-shaped rubber device filled with sperm-killing cream or jelly inserted into the vagina to cover the cervix.	95–98*
Foam	Sperm-killing foam inserted into the vagina shortly before intercourse.	97–98*
IUD (Intrauterine Device)	A plastic object inserted into the uterus. Discourages implantation of fertilized egg on uterine wall.	95–97*
Symptothermic Method	Combination of basal body temperature method and mucus observation (Billings method).	94–98.9*
Cervical Cap	Rubber cap which fits over the cervix and stays on by suction. Requires little cream or jelly.	92–98*
Lactation	Infant nursing suppresses ovulation.	91
The Pill	A combination of hormone-like drugs which suppresses the activity of a woman's ovaries.	90–98*
Depo-Provera	An injection of a progestogen-like drug which causes a woman to stop having periods. *(Note:* Despite the fact that Depo-Provera is not approved by the FDA as a method of birth control, physicians continue to prescribe it for this purpose.)	90–95*
Condom	Rubber sheath which covers the penis and catches semen.	90

(continued)

Method	Description	% Effectiveness
Billings Method	Requires total abstinence from sexual activity during a woman's fertile time. Based on recognition of the difference between fertile and nonfertile mucus.	80.6
Withdrawal	Practice of withdrawing the penis from the vagina before ejaculation.	80–90*
Rhythm (Calendar)	Predicting a woman's fertile time based on the length of her cycle.	79
Suppository	Solid sperm-killing "tablet" which melts when inserted into the vagina.	75–80*
Douching	Rinsing sperm from the vagina immediately after coitus by flushing with water or various solutions.	60

Methods with Limited Research

Method	Description	Possible % Effectiveness
Astrological	Predicting a woman's fertile time based upon coincidence of the relationship of the sun and moon with the time a woman was born. The woman must abstain from coitus 2½ days before and 2½ days after her fertile time. When the predicted fertile time does not coincide with other signs of ovulation, she must abstain also. The high effectiveness of this method results from the relatively few times when a woman can have coitus.	97.7
Lunaception	Based upon the idea that a certain hormone produced during darkness prevents an egg from developing. Women using this method must sleep in total darkness except for days 14, 15 and 16 of their cycles.	Never studied as a sole method of birth control.

* The reported range in percentage of effectiveness for some methods is due to the fact that the results of several different studies were used.

8 • Menstrual Extraction

Through working for abortion reform in the early 1970s, the early self-help clinic in Los Angeles became acquainted with the new, gentler suction method of removing the uterine contents—a method which was to revolutionize abortion technique. Out of this work they evolved the technology for removing a woman's flow, on a monthly basis or less often, and called it menstrual extraction.

They unearthed articles in Russian and Chinese medical journals showing hand-operated vacuum equipment and recommending the procedure for contraceptive purposes. They were aware of research in the United States on early-termination aspiration abortion without cervical dilation and with the use of a large syringe attached to a flexible plastic cannula (similar to a soda straw) or a portable foot pump.

The group found that menstrual extraction was not difficult to learn and that the introduction of a sterile four-millimeter cannula into the uterus was not traumatic because it did not require that the cervix be dilated. There was no cutting or scraping, so simple sterile procedures were sufficient; anesthetics were not necessary; and the suction was sufficient to extract all or most of a woman's flow in around 20 to 30 minutes.

The discovery that almost any woman could learn the technique of menstrual extraction was accompanied by the discovery of several obvious and very practical uses for it. Women could free themselves of heavy, crampy periods, or avoid having a period if it would interfere with travel, vacation or perhaps an athletic event, and could extract the contents of the uterus if there was the possibility of unwanted pregnancy.

Although menstrual extraction evolved out of work to make abortion safe and legal, the 1973 Supreme Court decision changed the group's primary interests to research of the method. They did not expect that all women would use menstrual extraction as a backup when birth control failed. They were aware, however, that one or two menstrual extractions a year carry far less health risks than either an IUD or the Pill.

Menstrual extraction and early termination abortion are similar technically, but menstrual extraction is not performed in a medical setting. When done by an experienced group, it can be used simply as a home-care procedure by women wishing to gain knowledge about their bodies and menstrual cycles and to exert more direct control over their reproductive lives.

Although prior discussion with her doctor as to her intention in using this particular technique is not absolutely necessary, having a physician available, should any medical questions arise, would further increase the safety of the procedure.

Menstrual extraction can be done in a woman's home or a self-help group's meeting place and the woman having her flow extracted controls all aspects of the procedure. Women generally learn the technique by participating in groups with more experienced women, first observing and then having their own menstrual extractions. Although the rudimentary aspects of the procedure can be learned in a few weeks, the knowledge and skill necessary to the reasonable safety of the procedure usually develop over a period of several months or even a year. Without this body of knowledge, the isolated woman, who generally has little or no familiarity with her own body, is risking the dangers commonly associated with self-abortion.

One frequent objection to menstrual extraction is a fear that the introduction of a cannula into the uterus will cause infections or other complications. Over the past decade, hundreds of women doing menstrual extraction in the United States and in other countries have reported that they do not have more or fewer infections than other women and have noted that the passage of a very small cannula into the uterus does not appear to have any effect on a woman's ability to carry a future pregnancy. It would seem, however, that the primary reason for this excellent safety record is the rigorous selection process any group doing menstrual extraction follows and the care with which the procedure is carried out. Women who have a tendency toward infection probably should not elect to have menstrual extraction. If they do, they take extra precautions. Sometimes a woman who is highly motivated but has a very sensitive cervix chooses to tolerate the additional discomfort in order to have an extraction.

Menstrual extraction should not be viewed as an attempt to avoid menstruation or short-circuit natural functions. It is a means for a woman to exert influence over changes in her body which she could not control before, in order to eliminate occasional discomfort or inconvenience or an unwanted pregnancy.

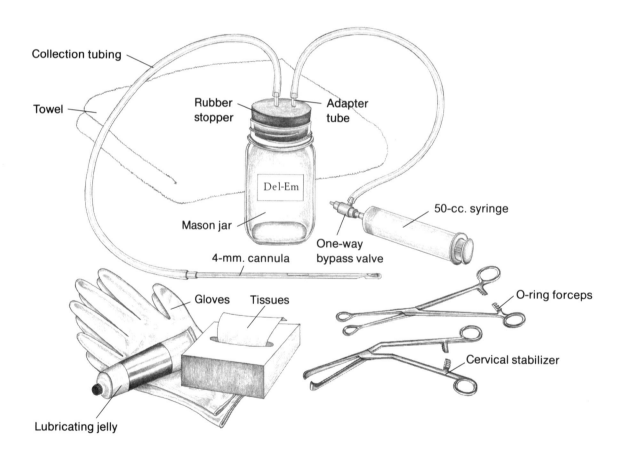

Collection tubing

Towel

Rubber stopper

Adapter tube

Del-Em

Mason jar

50-cc. syringe

4-mm. cannula

One-way bypass valve

Gloves Tissues

O-ring forceps

Cervical stabilizer

Lubricating jelly

8–1 Menstrual extraction equipment

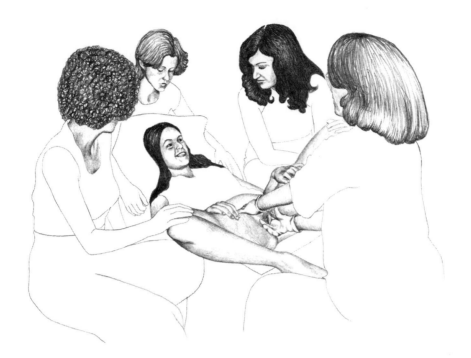

8–2 A woman having a uterine size check before menstrual extraction

8-1 Lorraine Rothman, one of the original members of the group which developed menstrual extraction, invented the Del-Em. After years of being a housewife, raising four children and numerous pets and working around her husband's biology lab, finding the components she needed was easy. She took a Mason jar from her pantry, a large stopper, some aquarium tubing and a 50-cc. syringe. She made inquiries at industrial supply houses and found a one-way bypass valve, which prevents air from returning once it has passed through. The total cost was just a few dollars, it worked, and anyone could make one. A kit similar to this one is currently being marketed for use in physician's offices. This illustration shows the basic supplies and equipment needed for menstrual extraction.

Many women report that their best experiences with menstrual extraction have taken place six weeks after their last period, give or take a week. However,

we know of menstrual extractions that have been done with complete safety and success up to eight or nine weeks after the last period. If the group has been doing self-examination consistently, they will be very familiar with the size and placement of the uterus and there will be much less chance of miscalculations.

8-2 The menstrual extraction usually takes place on the first day of a woman's *expected* period or several hours after her period starts. It can be done in comfortable surroundings, often in the woman's home. One or more experienced women in the group do a uterine size check to determine the size and position of the uterus, so that the group does not find itself dealing with a more advanced pregnancy than they are prepared for. Such a case could result in an incomplete extraction, which usually involves resorting to medical personnel who have access to the necessary equipment and skills to complete the procedure.

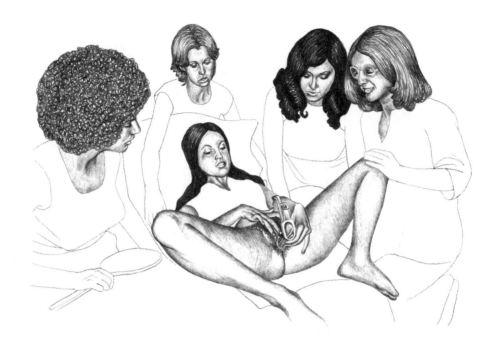

8–3   A woman inserting her speculum

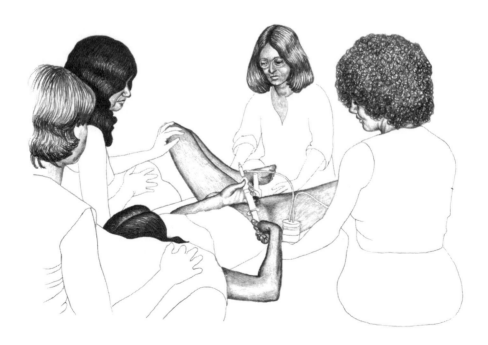

8–4   The woman who is having the extraction pumping
      the Del-Em

Wearing a surgeon's plastic glove, one woman inserts her index and middle fingers into the vagina. Pressing down on the abdomen just above the pubic hairline, she can feel the outline of the uterus between her hands. In early pregnancy, the uterus is usually the size of an unshelled walnut, and firm.

8-3 The woman who is having the extraction then inserts her own speculum and checks her cervix with a mirror. Then the other members of the group check it also. If she is pregnant, her cervix might very well be puffy and have a bluish tint. This change usually occurs in the first three months of pregnancy.

It is very important to the group to have information about the woman's menstrual cycle and her past experiences with menstrual extraction, irritations or infections or signs of pregnancy. Although the whole group should evaluate this information before proceeding, the final decision to proceed is always left to the woman who is having the extraction, provided she is sufficiently familiar with the technique to evaluate the information.

8-4 The next step is to pump up the vacuum in the Del-Em. Some women prefer to have the vacuum established before the cannula is inserted and this can be done by pinching the tube attached to the valve. Others prefer the suction to be built up slowly after the cannula is inserted into the uterus. If the woman decides to use the stabilizer, which looks like a pair of tweezers, it is attached to the cervix at this point. The stabilizer is used to keep the cervix from moving.

8-5 The cannula is now inserted carefully through the cervical canal into the woman's uterus. With the size four or five cannula, there is normally no need for dilation (stretching of the canal). The woman holding the cannula will feel it pass through the inner cervical opening and know the cannula tip is in the uterus.

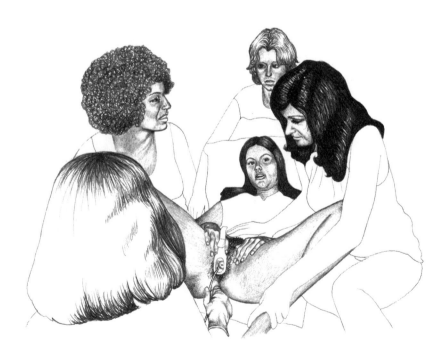

8-5   A self-helper inserting the cannula

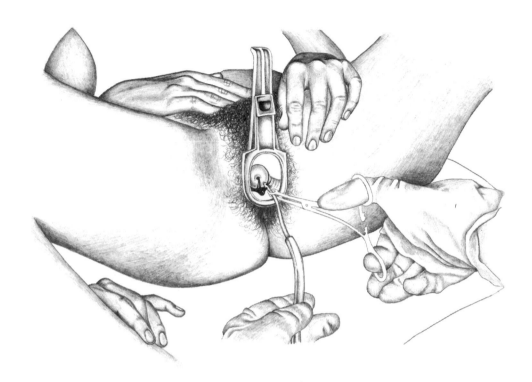

8–6 A woman holding the cannula with O-ring forceps

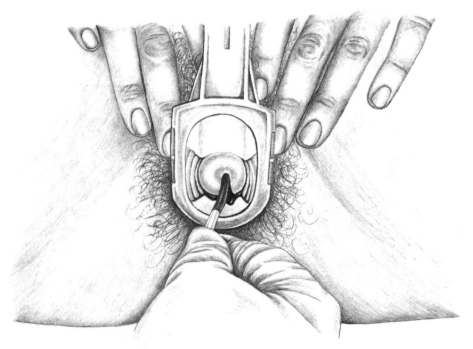

8–7 The cannula inserted into the uterus

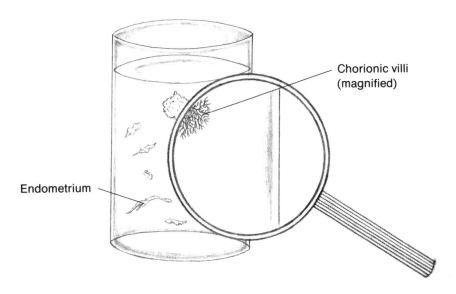

Chorionic villi
(magnified)

Endometrium

8–8   Chorionic villi in a glass

8-6 If the cannula does not go in easily, it is helpful to grasp it with the O-ring forceps to give it more stability.

8-7 When the cannula is in the uterus, the woman doing the extraction turns the cannula first in a clockwise direction, then in the opposite direction, and moves it forward and back as well, to make sure she is picking up all of the uterine material.

The woman having the extraction should always be in control. If her cramps are too heavy or if she feels too uncomfortable, she can ask that the extraction be stopped.

8-8 If a pregnancy has been interrupted, it is important that the extraction be complete. This can usually be determined by the woman, who will feel the stronger cramping that indicates the emptied uterus is contracting down to its usual size. The woman holding the cannula will usually notice a difference also. The cannula is harder to move in and out, and the interior of the uterus, which at first felt smooth, feels

rough, something like a washboard, when it is empty. The contents of the uterus—blood, clots or small bits of tissue—are examined in a shallow dish or glass. If chorionic villi, the yellowish material with branchlike structures which is the beginning of the placenta, are present, then it is a good sign that the menstrual extraction ended the pregnancy.

After menstrual extraction in which the woman was pregnant, the group stays in phone contact. If the woman thinks that she is still pregnant, the group may decide to repeat the procedure. In those rare instances when there are any signs of an infection, such as fever or discharge, heavy bleeding or pain and tenderness in the pelvic area, she must consult a physician immediately to obtain antibiotics since untreated uterine infections can be quite severe. She will know that the menstrual extraction was complete if the signs of pregnancy are gone with a few days and any minor cramping or bleeding has disappeared.

A NEW VIEW

The photographs in the color section represent the incredible variety of healthy women's genitals. They show some common vaginal conditions and the dynamic changes that occur throughout the menstrual cycle. These pictures are all of healthy women, and although they represent a fairly wide cross section, you should not be surprised if you look different from any picture you see here.

These photos were selected from more than a thousand taken of women from all over the United States and represent a variety of life styles and ethnic backgrounds, but we included a notation about ethnicity only when it seemed relevant to a specific point in a photograph.

To date, there has been scant research done by medical scientists on the menstrual cycle. Many of the photographs of cervixes are from a menstrual cycle study conducted by nine women at the Feminist Women's Health Centers in 1975, which greatly increased our knowledge about healthy changes during the menstrual cycle. Three of the nine participants' cervixes are shown here. In addition to daily photographs, the women made 36 different observations of daily changes in the appearance of the cervix, vagina and clitoris; the amount, color and texture of secretions; and recorded outside factors which they felt might influence their cycle.*

The brief health background for each woman is included, where it is relevant, to illustrate the range of experience the women have had with childbirth, abortion, birth control, sex and vaginal conditions. Although some of the information may not seem important, all of it does, in fact, have a bearing on that woman's condition. For example, for the pictures of the cervix, we attempted to include the precise day of the woman's cycle, because the appearance of the cervix changes from day to day. A woman's age is given to illustrate the point that the appearance of the cervix is *not* dependent upon age.

Through the photographer's lens, every feature of the cervix, vagina and clitoris stands out. So do certain other features, like the outline of the speculum, which often appears as a circle of light. The particular angle of the cervix and the color variations from picture to picture may be more the result of the photographic process than of something different or unusual about the cervix itself. The many different shots of the cervix illustrate the range of normal appearance and a number of common conditions which healthy women have.

The photos of the clitoris show its visible features in a way that should help you identify the different parts and to see that you are in no way unusual.

The photos in "Changes During the Menstrual Cycle" from the menstrual cycle study show the continuous and very distinct changes that occur throughout a woman's cycle, contrasted with the relative lack of change when a woman is on the Pill.

In the early stages of this project, self-helpers were taking photographs of their cervixes and vaginas with an instant camera. These photographs were very useful, but they did not reproduce well and color quality was undependable. Then they met filmmaker Sylvia Morales, who had never done any medical photography but was interested in experimenting with techniques that would enable women to have more information about their bodies.

Sylvia had to assemble her own equipment and try a variety of techniques in order to get lifelike color photos of the inside of the vagina. Her primary concern was to avoid any irritation or injury to the women who posed for the photographs. The most difficult problem was the heat of the flash, and in order to make sure that it caused no irritation to the cervix and mucous membranes of the vagina, she had to resort to a telephoto lens and work farther away.

The first series of Sylvia's photographs were exceptionally beautiful—so beautiful, in fact, that they made the inside of the vagina look like another world and detracted from the informational aspect of the photos. Therefore, she modified her technique to make them more straightforward and informative.

---

* The results of this study were presented by Suzann Gage at The Menstrual Cycle, an Interdisciplinary Nursing Research Conference, on June 28, 1977, at the College of Nursing, University of Illinois.

This woman is 19 years old. She started having periods when she was 13. She has no children and has had one abortion. She is not having a menstrual cycle because she is taking birth control pills.* She has intervals of bleeding from drug withdrawal that last approximately five days. There is no significant difference in the appearance of her cervix from one day to the next, due to the fact that the Pill is suppressing the normal menstrual cycle.

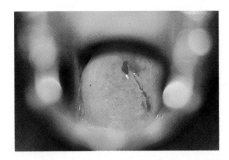

DAY 1. Day 23 of the Pill Cycle (sugar pill). Note the small amount of bleeding from withdrawal of the drug.

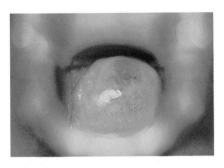

DAY 4. Day 26 of the Pill Cycle (sugar pill). Many women who take the Pill notice that their cervixes tend to be darker in color.

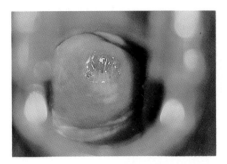

DAY 14. Day 8 of the Pill Cycle. Her squamocolumnar junction is visible, but does not seem to change much throughout her cycle.

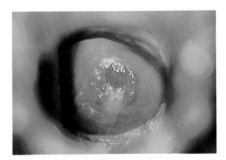

DAY 23. Day 17 of the Pill Cycle. Her cervix looks the same as it did on day 14.

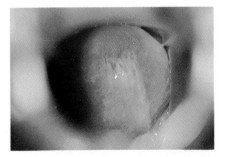

DAY 28. Day 22 of the Pill Cycle (sugar pill). She has a whitish secretion coming out of the os. This is the last day before breakthrough bleeding begins.

*The Pill Cycle: A woman takes a pill each day for 21 days. During this time most women do not have bleeding. Then she stops taking pills for seven days, or takes sugar pills instead. Within the next day or two (day 22 or so) most women get breakthrough bleeding which is really drug withdrawal bleeding that results from abruptly discontinuing the hormonelike drug contained in the Pill.

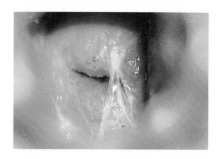

This woman, in her twenties, has had one child and one abortion and uses the diaphragm for birth control. The stringy mucus called "fertile mucus" is clear, but often mixes with whitish vaginal secretions. The openness of her os indicates that it is around the time of ovulation. The raised red spots near her cervix, like little blisters, occur frequently when she ovulates or is near her period. They come and go and she does not worry about them.

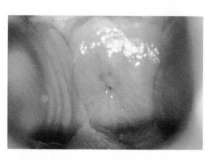

This woman's cervix has a few small red blotches near the os and you can see a clear mucus secretion coming out. Her vaginal wall, right next to the cervix, has a ripply texture. She is six weeks pregnant.

This woman, age 29, is on day 17 of her cycle. She has one child and has had one abortion. She uses the diaphragm for birth control and has not had sex recently. She thinks that the whitish, bubbly secretion on and around her cervix is possibly from a slight bacterial infection.

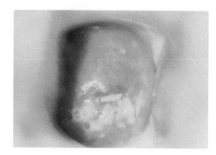

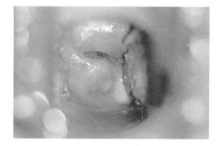

This woman's os is open and a creamy, whitish secretion is coming out. On each side, her vaginal walls appear to have a bumpy texture. The light-colored patches on the cervix are cysts which do not seem to give her any trouble. She has had four births, one miscarriage and one abortion (a D and C) and is 43 years old.

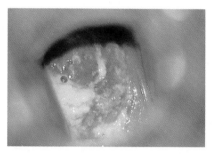

The secretion covering the cervix in this picture is white and clumpy. This woman typically has a lot of secretions and this secretion, a mixture of mucus and cast-off cells, is completely healthy. In appearance, it could be mistaken for a yeast condition, but it lacks the other characteristics of yeast, a yeasty odor or irritation of the vagina or clitoris. This photo was taken the day before her period was due. Note how dark the cervix is. Also, her cervix was cauterized by cryosurgery a year before and has had this irregular texture ever since.

This 21-year-old woman is on day 25 of her menstrual cycle. Although she thought she probably ovulated on day 20, her os is still open and clear mucus can be seen in it. She also has a very noticeable squamocolumnar junction. She has had no births or abortions. The white, creamy pool of secretions under her cervix is partly from a slight bacterial infection.

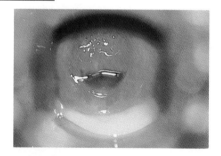

This woman is 23 years old and has had three abortions, one of which was done two-and-a-half weeks before this picture was taken. Her cervix does not look any different because of her recent abortion. Her cervix faces upward, indicating that her uterus is tilted backward, a perfectly normal position. This is called a "retroverted" uterus. She has some irritation on the cervix which does not bother her.

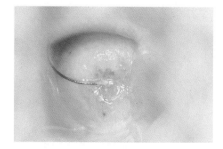

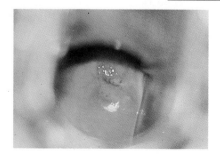

This woman is 28 years old and sexually active. She has had two children, which probably accounts for the shape of her os, and two miscarriages.

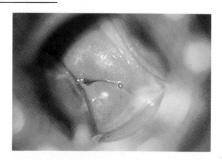

In this photo, an IUD string can be seen coming out of the os. The whitish part of the string at the os is where bacteria have gathered, like pus in an infection. This woman's IUD is a Dalkon Shield, a type that has been removed from the market in the U.S. because of the number of deaths and severe infections associated with it. (It is now recommended that every woman who has a Dalkon Shield have it removed.) She is 31 years old. The red spots above her os are irritations commonly seen on the cervixes of women who have IUDs.

9 • Feminist Abortion Care

Perhaps because of a long period of illegality, abortion has been greatly mystified and shrouded in myth. One prevailing myth is that early abortion is a surgical procedure. Another is that abortion is very dangerous, especially after the first three months. A particularly persistent misconception is that a woman must have a saline abortion—an induced miscarriage—after 15 weeks of pregnancy. Another myth is that after several abortions, a woman will have trouble carrying a pregnancy to term. Or that abortion is a painful, emotionally traumatic experience for most women.

Since before the 1973 Supreme Court decision making abortion in the first three months of pregnancy a decision between a woman and her doctor and making abortion from three to six months legal, but regulated by the states, feminists, abortion activists and committed physicians have worked to simplify and demystify the process of ending an unwanted pregnancy. The procedure they have developed is by far the safest and least traumatic available. It simplifies cumbersome medical routines and eliminates unnecessary requirements, so that having an abortion is more like going to the dentist than like having one's appendix removed.

An early-termination abortion is one that is performed up to about 14 weeks from the first day of the last menstrual period, or about 12 weeks from the time you became pregnant. Since your tissues are not cut and general anesthesia is unnecessary, early abortion is not surgery. Some women know that they are pregnant almost immediately and choose to have an abortion even before a pregnancy test would be accurate. Although most clinics and physicians prefer to wait until you have had a positive pregnancy test, the procedure, called a uterine aspiration, is available and is exactly like an abortion. Afterwards, pregnancy can be confirmed by laboratory examination of the uterine contents. (Most women can have a positive pregnancy test about two weeks after they miss their period, although there is a blood test that accurately detects pregnancy eight to ten days after conception.)

9-1 In a vacuum aspiration abortion, the contents of the uterus are suctioned out through a flexible plastic tube (a cannula) about the size of a soda straw. This normally takes about two or three minutes. During the procedure, you usually experience some cramping, which varies greatly from woman to woman, that comes from dilation of the cervix and from the muscular uterus closing back down to its normal size.

Since the procedure is so short, general anesthetic is not necessary, and is usually not offered in clinics.

In women-controlled clinics, the abortion itself is carefully designed to be as nontraumatic as possible. The smallest possible instruments are used. Since

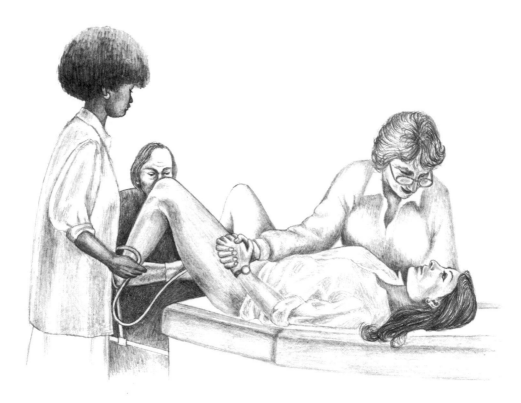

9–1 A woman having an early suction abortion

pain and trauma are the result of rapid, forceful stretching of the cervical canal, using a flexible cannula of the smallest possible size greatly reduces the pain and likelihood of injury. Another important factor in minimizing discomfort is the gentleness and skill of the abortionist.

The quality of a woman's abortion experience varies greatly in clinics, hospitals and doctors' offices. The best chance you have for safe, respectful care is in a clinic, particularly one owned and run by feminists. In a relaxed atmosphere where clinic routines are centered on the woman, where the emphasis is on providing information rather than on judgmental counseling, you can have a less unpleasant experience. A further advantage of a clinic abortion is that the abortion technicians are usually very experienced and highly skilled, much more so than a gynecologist who does just a few abortions each month.

There are a few possible complications of an early abortion. A few women develop uterine infections

when bacteria find their way into the uterus during or after the procedure or, occasionally, a small bit of retained tissue can become infected. Most hospitals require that all women take antibiotics to guard against the small chance of infection. (Only about two percent of women do develop infections and some individual clinics have a much lower rate.)

Another complication is an incomplete abortion. With a well-trained, skilled abortionist, this does not happen very often. When it does, a second, very short suctioning of the uterus can remove the remaining tissue.

By far the most infrequent complication is a uterine perforation, which happens when an instrument passes through the wall of the uterus. With a highly trained technician and the use of flexible plastic instruments, this is extremely rare.

The most progressive abortion clinics perform D and E (dilation and evacuation) abortions up to the eighteenth week of pregnancy under local anesthetic.

Between 18 and 20 weeks, women usually have to have the procedure done in a hospital, but can still have the D and E.

In some communities there are technicians who have done many, many procedures and have reached a high level of skill, so that they can do the D and E procedure through 24 weeks of pregnancy with greater relative safety than the saline procedure at the same number of weeks. The D and E after 20 weeks requires the insertion of a larger number of laminaria into the cervix, and sometimes they are even put in on two successive days before the abortion.

The later D and E abortion is quite similar to the vacuum aspiration. One difference is that the cervix is dilated with small sticks of seaweed called laminaria, which are inserted into your cervix the day before the procedure. Another difference is that the physician uses forceps to remove the tissue and fetal parts which are too large to pass through the cannula.

Many physicians also use a sharp metal instrument called a curette to scrape out the uterine contents (the traditional D and C). Others only use the curette to check at the end of the procedure to see if there is any tissue remaining in the uterus.

The D and E has the same types of risks as a suction abortion, although the chances of complication increase each week the pregnancy advances and there are some specific risks with D and E abortions as well. The two most common are tearing of the cervix and heavy bleeding or hemorrhage. These are rare complications, however, and their frequency varies a good deal according to the skill of the abortionist.

Many women believe that general anesthesia is necessary for an abortion after 12 weeks, but some clinics offer the choice of a local anesthetic, which is an injection into the cervix. The general anesthetic is only given in the hospital, and women who choose it face the same risks as anyone who has general anes-thetic. They also have a longer recovery period. The only thing that general anesthesia guarantees is that you will not feel anything *during* the abortion. Many women experience very painful cramps upon waking up from the anesthetic.

In most places, after about 20 weeks, saline (salt) abortion, or induced miscarriage, is the standard procedure. A solution of sterile salt water is injected into the uterus, which kills the fetus and irritates the uterine lining, thus causing a miscarriage. Many physicians still maintain that a saline abortion is the only appropriate procedure between 16 and 20 weeks, although the complication rate is higher for the saline than for the D and E.

Although the U.S. Supreme Court has said that every woman has the legal right to have an abortion up to the twenty-fourth week of pregnancy, its availability varies throughout the country. Women in rural areas have to travel great distances and, because of an amendment to the federal budget which prohibits the use of federal funds to pay for abortions for Medicaid recipients, in most states poor women are finding them totally unavailable. This amendment, sponsored by Congressman Henry Hyde of Illinois, a powerful member of the Right-to-Life movement, was opposed by women's health groups, the women's movement and many groups which support women's rights to control their own reproduction. In mid-1980, by a narrow five-to-four majority, the Supreme Court ruled in favor of the Hyde Amendment, thereby denying poor women access to safe abortion care. Many women will be forced to have children they do not want or to resort to illegal abortions, which are cheaper. It is a tragedy that when abortion is legal and available to women who have money, it is not possible for all women to receive safe, up-to-date procedures in a supportive environment.

9-2 This illustration shows the uterus eight to nine weeks after the beginning of the last normal menstrual period. The abortionist is holding a stabilizer with the left hand and the flexible plastic cannula with the right. The uterine contents will be suctioned out through the cannula which is attached to a plastic tubing and a vacuum bottle.

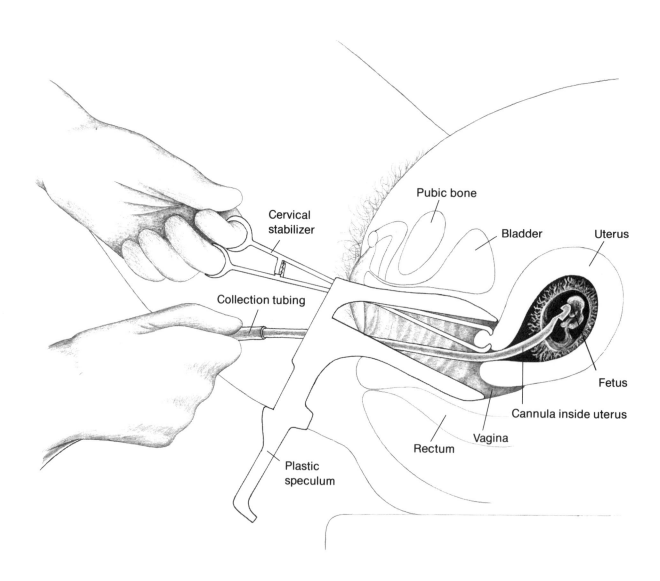

Cervical stabilizer

Collection tubing

Plastic speculum

Pubic bone

Bladder

Uterus

Fetus

Cannula inside uterus

Vagina

Rectum

9-2   An early suction abortion

9-3 In two to three minutes, the uterus is empty and has closed down again to its prepregnant size. A plastic vaginal speculum should be used instead of a weighted metal speculum, which weighs up to five pounds and is used in most doctors' offices and in hospitals.

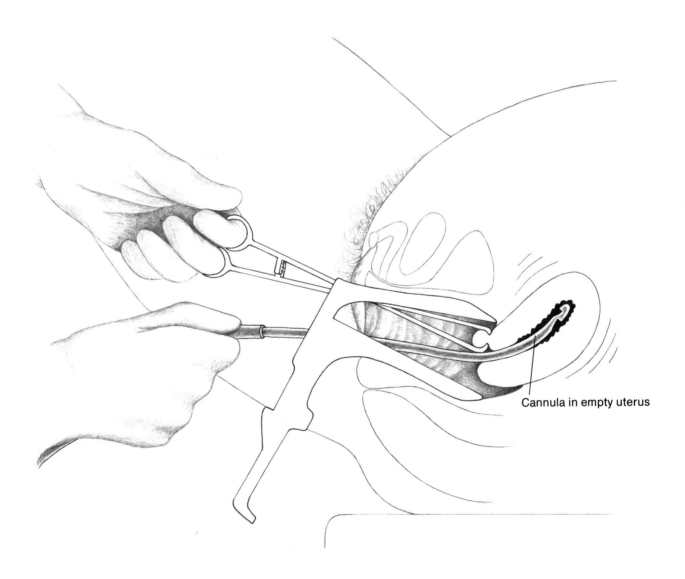

Cannula in empty uterus

9-3   An early suction abortion completed

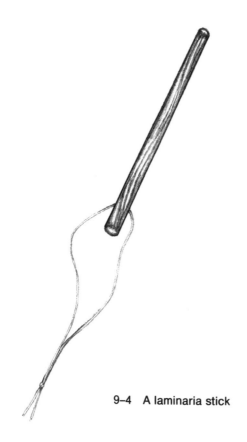

9–4   A laminaria stick

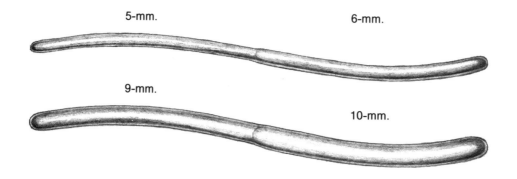

5-mm.   6-mm.

9-mm.

10-mm.

9–5   Dilators of different sizes

9-4 Laminaria are sticks of sterile seaweed about the size of kitchen matches. Up to five or six are inserted into a woman's cervix at least six hours, and often overnight, before an abortion. The sticks swell to about the size of a pencil by absorbing secretions from the cervix. This dilates the cervical canal slowly and gently and makes it unnecessary to use heavy metal dilators. Some women have cramps as the cervical canal opens, but the abortion procedure is shorter and therefore less uncomfortable.

Laminaria have long been used in Japan to dilate women's cervixes naturally.

9-5 These graduated dilators are used to open up your cervical canal so that a cannula can be inserted to suction out fluid and tissue. If you are about six to eight weeks pregnant, it is probably only necessary to use the five- to six-millimeter dilator. The largest dilator used up to about 12 weeks is a nine- to ten-millimeter dilator. After 12 weeks, laminaria are used instead of dilators.

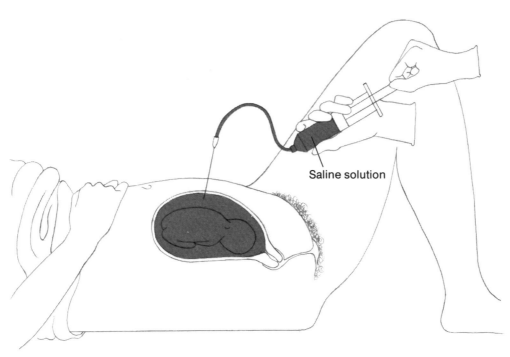

Saline solution

9–6 A saline abortion

9-6 A saline (salt solution) abortion is an induced miscarriage. Usually a little amniotic fluid is withdrawn from the uterus and replaced with about three to four cups of saline solution. The solution kills the fetus and causes the uterus to contract and expel it. The uterus contracts as it does in labor, so you go through a shortened version of labor, usually about six to eight hours.

The saline injection itself does not hurt; it is, at worst, uncomfortable and causes a feeling of fullness. A saline abortion, however, can be extremely upsetting experience, and just like labor, can be very painful. Nonetheless, many women still choose to have a saline procedure rather than to continue their pregnancies.

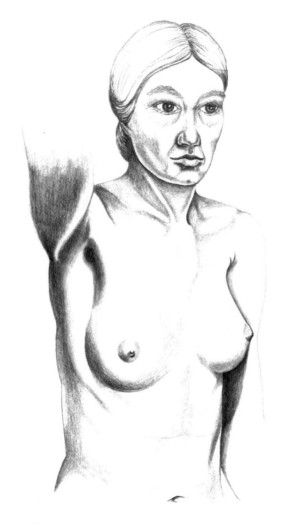

10–1   A view of a healthy woman's breasts

10 · Serious Health Problems: Surgery

Surgery is used for repair after disease or an accident, for treatment of certain conditions and as a diagnostic tool. For women, gynecological surgery is more frequent than any other kind, and quite a bit of it has been shown to be unnecessary—unnecessary because other forms of treatment (or even prevention) are available, or because, as in the case of drastic breast surgery, the surgery is not a particularly effective cure.

The types of major surgery that women are most concerned about are breast surgery and hysterectomy. These operations drastically alter the body and, in the case of complete hysterectomy, severely affect a woman's hormonal production, at least temporarily. Any woman who is faced with surgery wants to know that it is the best possible treatment with the least undesirable physical effects, and that she has made her choice based upon reliable, complete information.

When gynecological surgery is recommended, especially more radical operations like mastectomy, the removal of one or both breasts and associated structures, or hysterectomy, the removal of the uterus, tubes and ovaries, you need to be wary. Often these surgeries are recommended without solid reasons. For example, there is an alarming trend among U.S. physicians to do "prophylactic" hysterectomies—in other words, to remove the uterus *before* a disease condition shows up, on the statistical chance that one *might* develop. Our uteruses are also removed because many doctors think that once their childbearing function is

finished, they are prone to disease and that we have no more use for them at that point anyway. One third to one half of all hysterectomies are unnecessary!

One way to avoid unnecessary surgery is to seek a second opinion. If it differs considerably, or especially if it is the same, you may even want to get a third opinion. Although many women do seek second opinions, statistics reveal that physicians in the same profession tend to rubber-stamp initial opinions. One way to guard against this tendency is to seek the opinion of a physician in a different specialty. You might check the opinion of your gynecologist with an internist. Often, the result of another evaluation can be the option of a less drastic form of treatment, or the decision to adopt a wait-and-see strategy, if it is appropriate.

It has been standard medical practice to make a decision to perform major surgery based on the results of a biopsy (an examination of a tissue sample from a suspect tumor) which is evaluated while you are still under anesthesia. The Women's Health Movement has helped make it possible for a woman to assert her right to evaluate the results of her biopsy before consenting to major and perhaps debilitating surgery.

It is possible for a great deal of minor surgery, including some biopsies, to be done under a local anesthetic. You may prefer to be awake just so you will know exactly what is happening. Under these circumstances, drastic surgery cannot be performed without your consent. Others do not want to undergo the small definite risks that general anesthetic carries. Still others choose a local anesthetic because of the shorter recovery time. A local anesthetic is usually an injection of a painkiller into the affected area, and can be combined with a tranquilizer to further lessen sensation.

Any kind of surgery is traumatic and, of course, the better physical condition you are in, the faster recovery will be. Some women who are able to exercise and follow the most nutritious diet possible before surgery find that their recoveries are far quicker than predicted by their surgeons. Their experiences also indicate that strengthening muscles, especially around the affected area, seems to have a direct, positive effect on the speed of recovery.

Also, surgeons differ in their technical skills and in their care to use the least traumatic methods. Generally, it is worthwhile to make inquiries of anyone you know in the medical community, as it is often common knowledge there who the most- and least-skilled surgeons are. Recovery time and aftereffects can be dramatically different, depending on the skill of the surgeon.

Breast Surgery

Most of the lumps women find when doing breast self-examination are not cancerous. They could be cysts, fatty tumors, lymph nodes, or warty growths called papillomas which sometimes occur under the nipples. When a woman first finds a breast lump, her reaction is often fear and uncertainty. The first thing she can do to reassure herself is to evaluate the characteristics of the lump. If it is movable, if it hurts or is similar to any other mass in either breast, it is probably not dangerous. Cancerous lumps are usually painless, hard and difficult to manipulate. Cysts and benign tumors are usually self-contained and suspended in the breast tissue.

This preliminary check is not for the purpose of self-diagnosis. Rather, it is an important first step in arming yourself against the unfolding of an all-too-familiar scenario. Countless times, health workers have heard the story of how a woman rushes to her doctor in panic to be presented with a frightening range of possibilities. She then immediately packs her bag and checks herself into the hospital for diagnostic tests in the early morning hours of the next day. Ironically, the lump is hardly ever cancerous and could easily have been dealt with in the physician's office and this nightmare for a woman and her family could have been avoided.

The standard medical treatment for any tumor which has been identified as cancerous is surgery, and the more the better, based on the idea that it is necessary to get the cancer before it spreads.

In the 1890s, a doctor named Halsted developed the radical mastectomy and in the 1920s, on the basis of a very small study, it became the preferred surgery for dealing with breast cancer. In the past several years it has become apparent that the cure rate for radical mastectomy is not particularly good, possibly because by the time cancer develops in the breast, active cancer cells are harbored in other parts of the body, growing quickly or slowly, depending on unknown factors. Women who find that cancer is in the lymph nodes have few choices, but since the cure rate for radical mastectomy is no better than that for a simple or modified radical mastectomy, they might choose the less drastic surgery and supplement with radiation or chemotherapy, or a combination of both. If, as current cancer specialists suspect, cancer is a systemic disease, all measures which improve the body's resistance to disease generally may improve the length and certainly the quality of a woman's survival.

Increasingly, women are seeking out doctors who use either vitamin C therapy or Laetrile, a highly controversial anticancer drug, instead of resorting to surgery. Laetrile therapy is based on an entirely different theory about the origin and course of cancer and is not inconsistent with concepts presently being discussed in the medical establishment. Because research on Laetrile has been suppressed by the government and medically controlled institutions, considering the lack of success of surgical treatment and the claims for Laetrile's success given by many cancer victims, this option deserves serious consideration. A woman may have to travel to obtain Laetrile, since it is legal in only 23 states. Although radical mastectomy is still most physicians' preferred treatment, it is not preferred by women who know that its cure rate is no better than that of less scarring and mutilating treatment.

If you decide to consult your doctor about a lump, you will have a range of choices for diagnosis. (The doctor can't tell much by just feeling the lump either.) If a cyst is suspected, it can be aspirated or drained with a needle in the doctor's office using local anesthetic. But if the lump has the characteristics of a cancerous tumor, one of the several forms of X-ray diagnosis can be used: mammography (high-exposure X-rays); xeroradiography (low-exposure X-rays); thermography (detects heat from fast-growing cysts); or transillumination (strong light to illuminate dense masses in the breast). The use of mammography, xeroradiography and thermography has been the subject of a heated controversy, and it is now recommended that they not be used as a routine diagnostic tool for women under the age of 50, and over 50 only when there is significant risk of cancer. In fact, recent information reveals that repeated exposure to low-level radiation in younger women may stimulate true cancers which were likely to remain dormant for a lifetime. In making the decision to have a mammography, women need to be exceedingly cautious. Reputable facilities have been discovered to use widely varying amounts of radiation—often many times the amount women need in routine screening (.007 rad—a unit used to measure radiation—is sufficient for an effective mammogram). It has also been noted that dosage emission is not just a matter of fancy new equipment; instead, it is dependent on proper maintenance and the skill of the technician who operates the machine.

It is also important to realize that these diagnostic tools alone are inadequate to confirm cancer. Only a surgical biopsy which removes the lump and makes it available for analysis over a period of days can give an accurate diagnosis and (with other tests) prognosis.

For women who find that a lump is cancerous, the choice of treatment is critical. Some cancerous lumps grow rapidly and some grow more slowly, and their location and size are extremely important considerations. The final determinant is a surgical biopsy which identifies the precise type of cells, combined with tests to determine if active cancer cells are also in the lymph nodes. Although the biopsy can often be taken under a local anesthetic, it is usually taken under a general, and the tissue is evaluated immediately. False positives have been known to result from such hurried analysis and this course of action has worked to the disadvantage of many women who have awakened from their biopsies to discover that they have no breast. Some researchers have suggested, in fact, that microscopic examination of the tissue is not always clear-cut and that the results may, in some cases, be debatable. Also, the one-step course of action gives a woman no time to consider her alternatives, which include surgery, radiation, chemotherapy, some combination of these, or vitamin C therapy or Laetrile. Critics see this one-step procedure as serving mostly the convenience of the physician and hospital staff. Physicians, however, contend that this one-step operation saves money and risk from additional anesthetic. Although you must sign a consent form if mastectomy is to immediately follow the biopsy result, you are often induced to do so on the basic of faulty or incomplete information about your choices.

One of the major drawbacks of radiation therapy is that radiation, in numerous forms, is known to cause cancer. In therapy, it can be applied externally from an X-ray machine, or can be implanted in or near a tumor in the form of capsules or needles. The radiation destroys cancer cells, but it also destroys normal red blood cells which are necessary to fight off infection. This treatment is often used in combination with surgery or chemotherapy.

Survival rates of women who have had radiation treatment have compared favorably with those of women who have had radical mastectomies. Radiologists feel that radiation therapy in combination with minimal surgery or local excision can result in a survival rate of at least five years for 80 to 90 percent of women with early breast cancer.

Chemotherapy generally refers to a wide variety of drugs which are used in the treatment of cancer. These drugs frequently work by poisoning cancer cells or by interfering with their division. Like radiation, chemotherapy also kills healthy cells. It also has many harmful effects and causes most people to feel very sick. Nausea, weight loss and the loss of hair are common results. Dosages must be carefully chosen and the recipients constantly monitored for damage to healthy cells or tissue. For these reasons, it seems important to choose a physician who has had a lot of experience with this type of treatment.

When a breast cancer is confirmed through a biopsy, the ovaries are sometimes removed as well as the breast, on the suspicion that the tumor is "estrogen dependent," that it, it is stimulated to grow by the body's natural estrogens. In the past, the decision to remove the ovaries was based on conjecture, but now there is an estrogen-receptor assay (ERA) test which can be done at the same time as a surgical biopsy. The test must be done within 15 minutes after removal of the tissue, and must be arranged for in advance. Many surgeons do not offer this test routinely, so you may need to request it. If the tumor is very small, it is not always possible to do the test, since one gram of malignant tissue is required

When a woman is fully aware of her condition and of her options, she can make a choice which she is most comfortable with and one which is best for her.

For women who are faced with extensive surgery like mastectomy or hysterectomy, support groups are now available to help make adjustments to changes in their lives which come about because of radical surgery or other drastic treatment.

10-1 *(page 136).* The breast tissue begins underneath the breasts and includes the breasts themselves, side and underarm tissue, a network of lymph nodes and pectoral muscles.

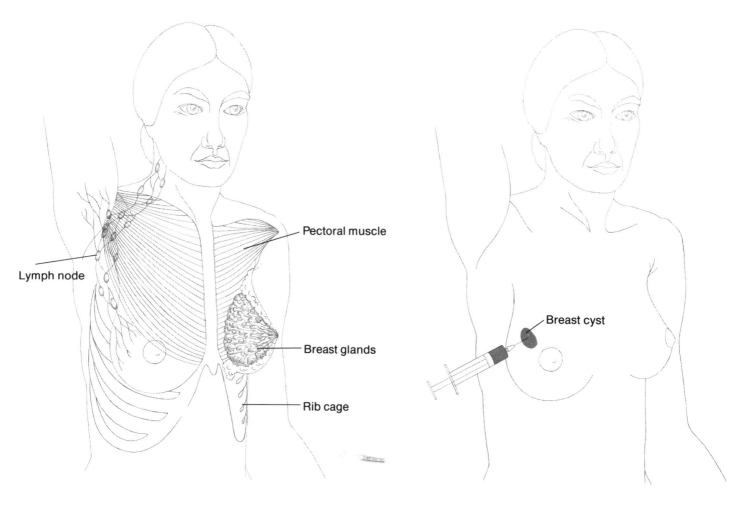

10-2 Different parts of the breasts which may be removed during surgery

10-3 Aspiration of a breast cyst

10-2 This illustration shows the underlying structures of the breast: the rib cage, pectoral muscles,
lymph nodes, fat and milk glands. These are the
structures affected by breast surgeries. In radical mastectomies, even the ribs are broken to get at the
glands behind the breast bone. The right breast
glands are transparent to show the entire pectoral
muscle.

10-3 A suspected breast cyst is aspirated with a
hollow needle and syringe and this can be done in a
doctor's office with or without local anesthetic. In this
simple procedure, the doctor pierces the skin with the
needle and finds the cyst beneath. If fluid is withdrawn, you can be sure that the lump is a cyst. When
all of the fluid is removed, the cyst usually collapses
and does not return.

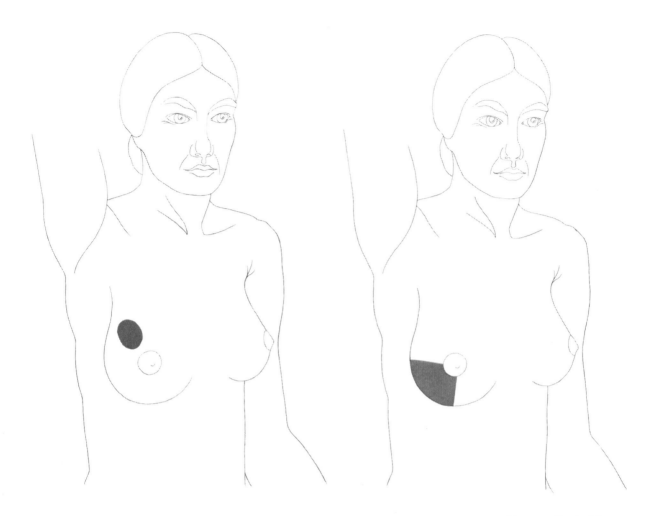

10–4 Lumpectomy: Tissue affected by removal of a lump

10–5 Segmental mastectomy: Tissue affected by removal of a lump and surrounding tissue

10-4 If you have a cancerous lump, you may be able to find a physician who will remove *only* the lump. The physician makes an incision from one to three inches long, removes the lump and surrounding tissue and sends it to the laboratory for examination. This procedure, called lumpectomy, can be done in a doctor's office under local anesthetic and is the one most preferred for removing noncancerous growths. If the lump is cancerous, its removal is often accompanied by radiation or other treatment.

10-5 A segmental mastectomy, also called partial mastectomy or wedge resection, removes the lump, the skin covering it and the breast tissue to the depth of the membrane that covers the chest muscles. This operation is only useful if the lump is small, self-contained and fairly close to the nipple. After the tissue has been removed, the breast can be reconstructed to its former shape at a later time if it is planned for before surgery. If the nipple is not disturbed, women who have this surgery can still breast-feed.

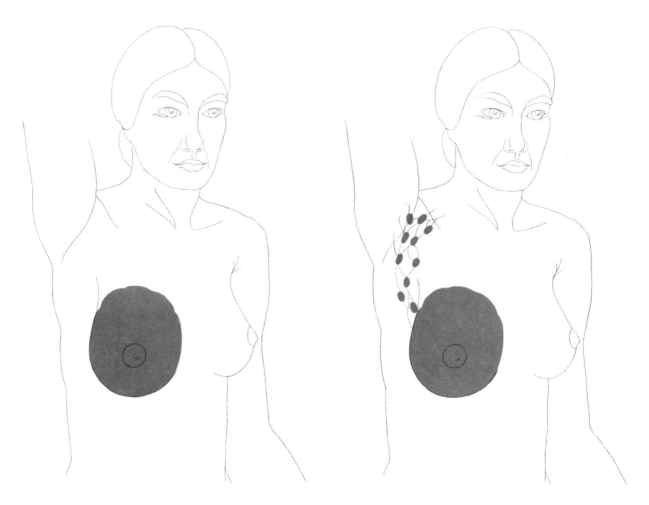

10–6 Simple mastectomy: Tissue affected by removal of breast tissue down to the muscles

10–7 Modified radical mastectomy: Tissue affected by removal of the breast and lymph nodes

10–6 In a simple mastectomy (also called a total mastectomy) only the tissues of the breast itself are removed down to the depth of the membrane covering the pectoral muscles. This might be combined with removing a sample of the lymph nodes in the armpit. Recovery from this surgery is usually fairly rapid. You might choose to have this procedure and combine it with radiation, chemotherapy or vitamin C therapy or Laetrile. Reconstruction is possible if it is arranged for prior to the initial surgery.

10–7 A modified radical mastectomy removes all of the breast and some surface lymph nodes. Little skin is removed, and because the chest and arm muscles are left intact, you have a better chance to regain the use of your arm and can often regain strength faster. Since lymph nodes filter fluid and remove bacteria or other harmful substances from the bloodstream, they are a vital part of the body's defense against infection. When all of the nodes are removed from your chest and underarm, you may be plagued with chronic swelling. Surgeons usually try to remove all tissue containing active cancer cells, but the cure rate for this surgery is roughly the same as for a radical or a simple mastectomy, and it is not always offered as an option.

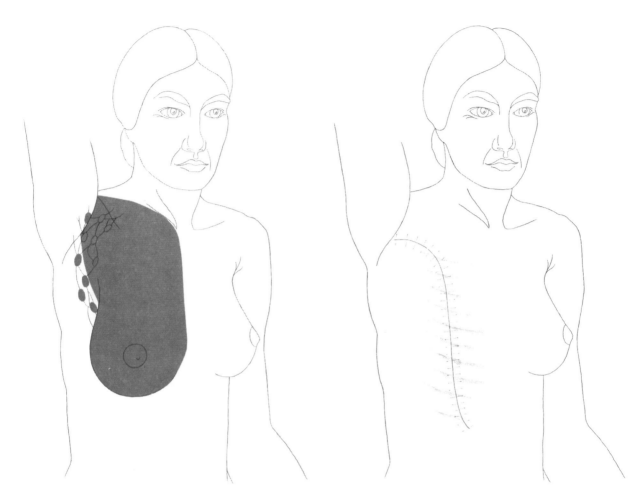

10-8 Radical mastectomy: Tissue affected by removal of the breast, lymph nodes and muscles

10-9 A scar from a radical mastectomy

10-8 A radical mastectomy is an intricate, time-consuming operation in which the skin, breast, lymph nodes and pectoral muscles are removed. It has many severe and long-lasting physical effects. Some women say that it takes as long as a year to recover fully, while others never feel the same again. They also experience higher mortality and have a higher risk of respiratory illness.

10-9 The aftereffects of radical breast surgery are, for many women, devastating. The most obvious result is the deep and extensive scarring. If many lymph nodes are taken, you are likely to experience swelling or infection in your arm, because there is no lymph system to filter fluids. You will never have your former strength again, because the pectoral muscles, which help in lifting, have been cut away. If many nerves are cut, you can feel a numbness in your arm and shoulder, although this eventually disappears in most cases. Since all of this surgery does not significantly increase most women's chances for survival, you might want to choose a less drastic procedure or a different form of treatment altogether, such as radiation, chemotherapy, which can be combined with the surgery, or more controversial but less drastic treatments, such as vitamin C therapy or Laetrile (which is becoming increasingly more available).

10–10   Burning closed the egg tubes for sterilization

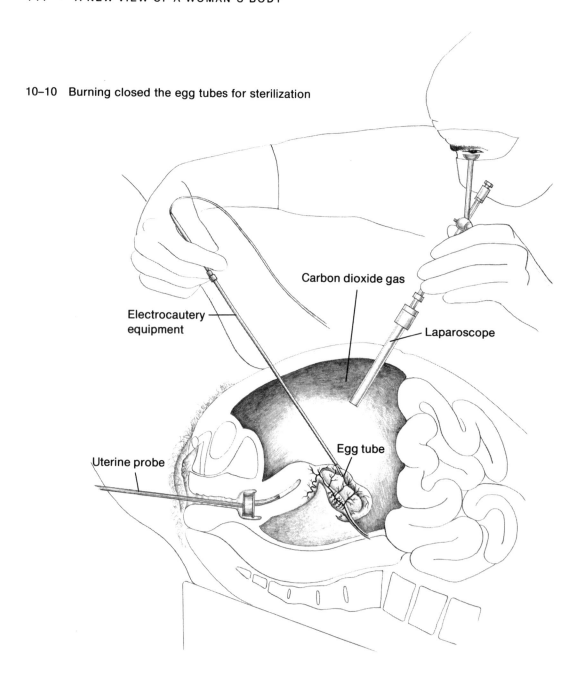

Electrocautery equipment

Carbon dioxide gas

Laparoscope

Uterine probe

Egg tube

10–10 "Band-Aid" surgery, or tubal ligation using a laparoscope to burn the tubes (commonly known as "having the tubes tied"), is in fact a major operation that usually requires a general anesthetic and heavy sedation afterward. The procedure is very painful and the recovery time is anywhere from a few days to a few weeks.

Laparoscopy is a surgical method of sterilization in which the egg tubes are either sewn or burned shut, severed or blocked by tiny plastic rings. In this procedure, your abdomen is filled with carbon dioxide gas so that the muscular abdominal wall will balloon

away from the uterus and tubes. A small incision is made in your belly button and a metal tube is inserted through the layers of fat and muscle. A laparoscope, an instrument which emits a heatless light, is then inserted through the tube. Another small cut is made just above the pubic hairline to allow the entrance of the instruments to cut, sew, burn or install the rings. In this illustration, the surgeon is burning the tube with a metal instrument attached to an electric current—a procedure called electrocautery.

As with abortions, women who have a local anesthetic tend to recover faster than women who have a

10–11 The dilation for a D and C

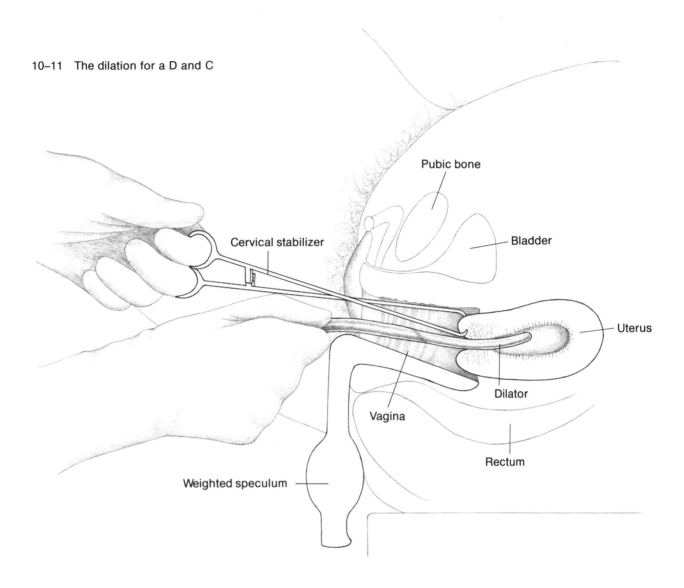

Pubic bone

Bladder

Cervical stabilizer

Uterus

Dilator

Vagina

Rectum

Weighted speculum

general anesthetic. This procedure is also used to remove a stray IUD from the abdominal cavity, to end a pregnancy in the tubes or to identify problems of infertility.

Numerous government-funded programs have forced women of color to be sterilized. In Los Angeles, California, ten women of Mexican descent sued physicians from Los Angeles County-University of Southern California Medical Center for sterilizing them without their full knowledge or consent. Native American women have been sterilized unknowingly in Indian Health Service Hospitals. Some family planning personnel have encouraged sterilization by minimizing the risks of the surgery when counseling women or when consulting for articles in the popular media. Government regulations, shaped by the protests of people of color and women's groups, now require a waiting period before a woman can get sterilization surgery on public funds, an effort to prevent further abuse.

10–11 The D and C (dilation and curettage) is the gynecological standby. It is used for everything: abortion, infertility, uterine infection, severe menopause symptoms, fibroids, heavy bleeding or diagnosis of cancer. A physician usually uses a heavy weighted speculum to open the vagina; she or he then attaches a stabilizer (like a long pair of tweezers) to the cervix and inserts successively larger metal rods through the cervical canal to stretch it enough to allow the entry of the curette.

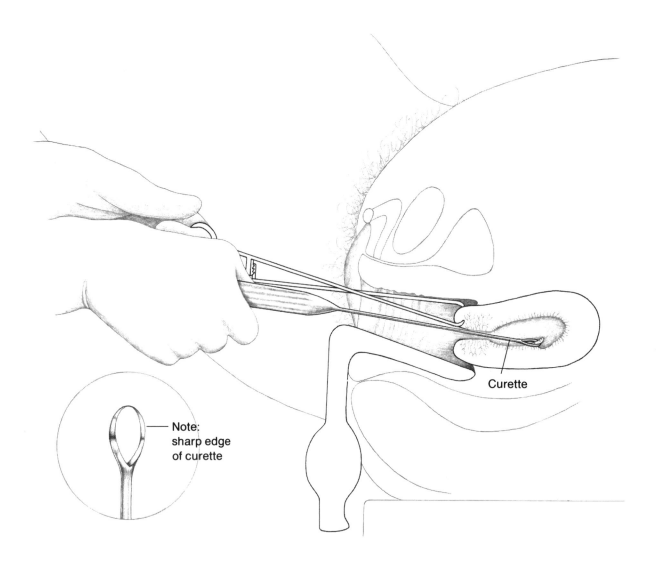

Note:
sharp edge
of curette

Curette

10–12   Curetting, or scraping away the uterine lining
during a D and C

10–12 A curette is a sharp metal instrument with a small looped end which is used to scrape away the uterine lining. In most of the cases for which a D and C is recommended for abortion, a vacuum aspiration is just as effective, has a lower risk and is far less traumatic.

A physician should have a strong justification for performing a D and C instead of vacuum aspiration.

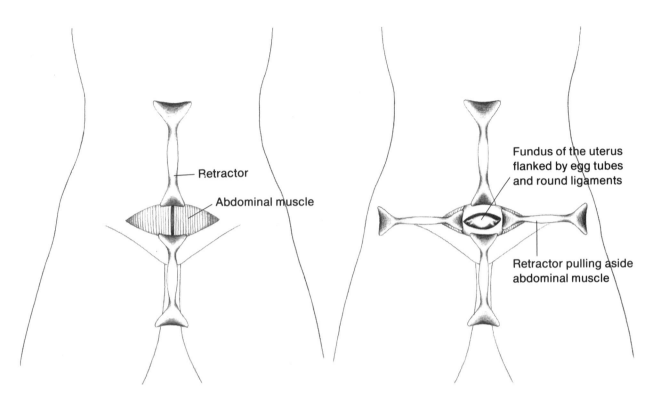

10–13 Step one in opening the abdominal wall for pelvic surgery

10–14 Step two in opening the abdominal wall

10-13 Laparotomy means a pulling back of the abdominal wall in order to perform surgery in the pelvic area. First, a small incision is made and the skin and muscles are retracted horizontally on each side of the incision with metal retractors.

10-14 Two other retractors are then used to pull back a second layer of muscle and tissue. This procedure is used for hysterectomy, retrieval of stray IUDs, removal of fibroids and ovarian egg-tube or bladder surgery.

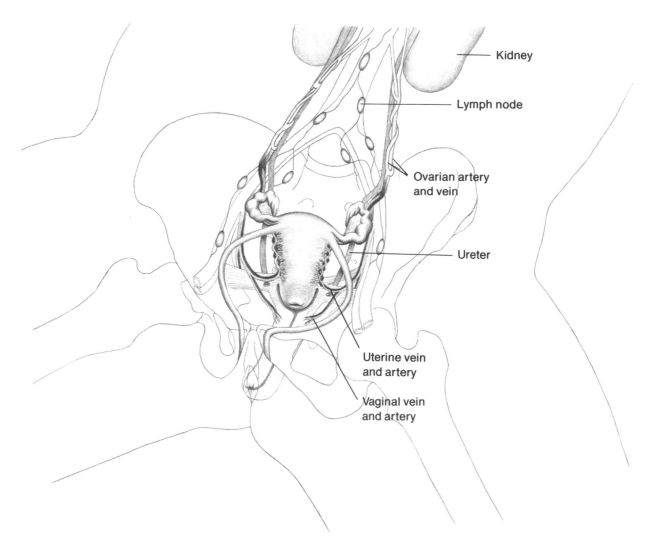

Kidney

Lymph node

Ovarian artery
and vein

Ureter

Uterine vein
and artery

Vaginal vein
and artery

10–15 The uterus before a hysterectomy (bladder is
not shown)

10–15 This illustration shows the cervix and uterus with ligaments and blood vessels, tubes and ovaries in their normal positions.

10–16 A simple complete hysterectomy is the removal of the uterus and cervix. A partial hysterectomy (not shown) leaves the cervix intact.

10–17 A radical hysterectomy is the removal of the uterus, tubes, ovaries, cervix, lymph nodes and vaginal tissue. Physicians often connect the uterus with reproduction alone instead of acknowledging that it also plays an integral part in sexual response. So when a physician tells you that you won't really need your uterus, you can tell him that indeed you might.

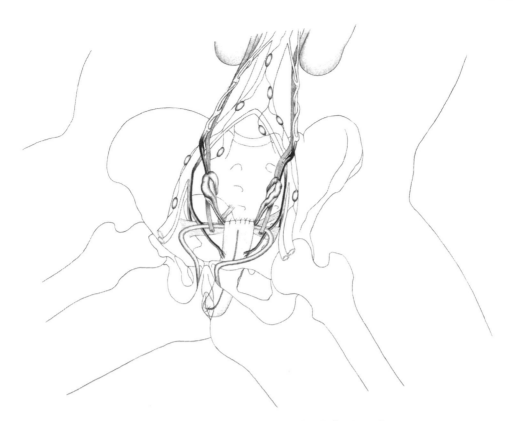

10–16   The pelvic area after a simple hysterectomy

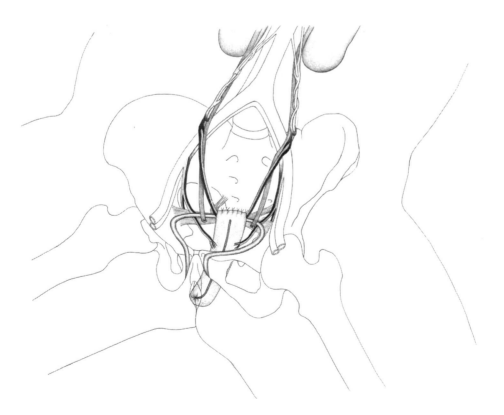

10–17   The pelvic area after a radical hysterectomy

10-18 Conization is one medical treatment for unusual-looking cells on the cervix (cervical dysplasia) or a suspected precancerous condition. Conization, which is the surgical removal of a cone-shaped core from the center of the cervix, is used for both diagnosis and treatment, especially if cancer is suspected, and a D and C is usually done at the time to determine if there are any cancerous cells in the uterus. Conization is also a treatment for chronic irritation of the cervix which is resistant to treatment, but it is an extremely drastic measure to take to remedy this condition.

The first step is to cut the cone-shaped core around the mouth of the cervix with a scalpel.

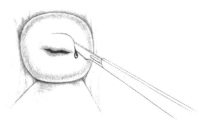

10-18   First step of a conization

10-19 The second step is to remove the core with an instrument called a tenaculum, which looks like a long pair of tweezers.

The complications from this surgical procedure are heavy bleeding or hemorrhage, infection, or uterine perforation if the instrument pokes through the uterine wall.

Since anywhere from one fourth to one half of the face of the cervix is removed, this operation can have significant effect on both the appearance and function of the cervix. Scar tissue can make the opening to the cervix much less elastic and the cervical canal weaker, which may increase the chances of miscarriage if a woman becomes pregnant.

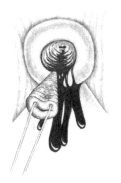

10-19   Second step of a conization

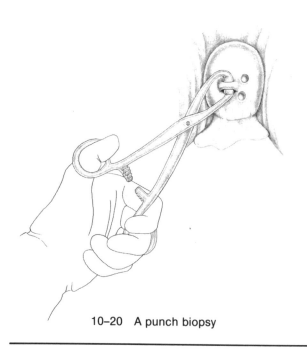

10-20   A punch biopsy

10-20 A punch biopsy, a simple, diagnostic procedure which is done in a doctor's office, is used to further check suspicious results from a Pap smear. Small bits of tissue are removed from the face of the cervix with an instrument that looks like a paper punch. The cervix is painted with an iodine solution before the tissue samples are taken. Since there are not a lot of nerve endings in the cervix, the procedure does not cause much pain, but it can cause cramping and sometimes a little bleeding.

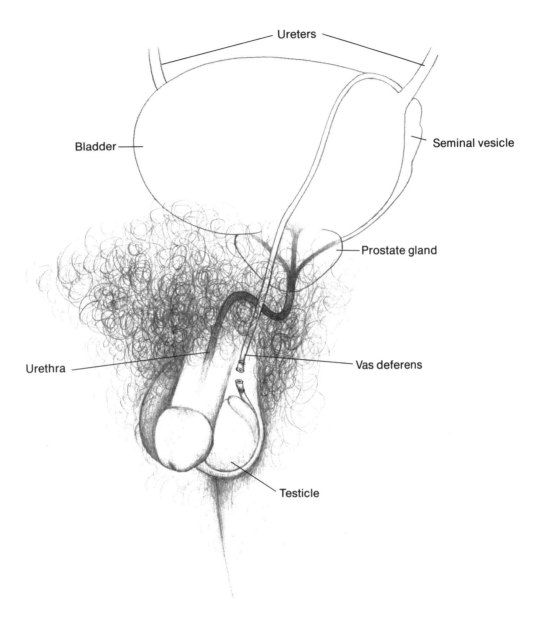

Ureters

Bladder

Seminal vesicle

Prostate gland

Urethra

Vas deferens

Testicle

10–21   The vas deferens after a vasectomy

10-21 Vasectomy is a safe, highly effective method of sterilization for men. It is an office procedure which has a low complication rate. One vas deferens, the tube through which the sperm travel through the prostate gland, is snipped just behind the testicles. The procedure is repeated for the other side. This prevents the sperm from reaching the prostate gland where it is mixed with seminal fluid. The tube is then tied, sewn or clipped, to prevent it from growing back.

The procedure can be done in an outpatient clinic.

The main objection men have to vasectomy is that, at this time, it is almost irreversible, but ironically, there have been cases where the vas deferens has grown back on its own. About one half to one third of men will develop antibodies to the sperm following vasectomy, but it is not known whether this leads to any health problems.

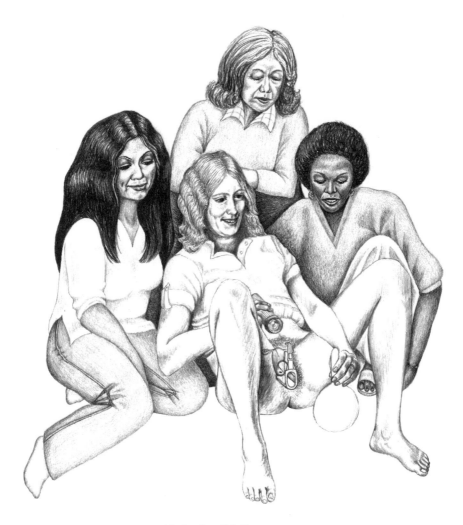

11-1 A self-help group

11 · A Self-Help Clinic

11-1 A self-help clinic can happen any time, anywhere women get together to share the techniques of self-examination and to discuss their health. The focus is on sharing experiences and information, on exploring normal, healthy differences and common health concerns about menstruation, vaginal conditions, birth control, hormones and menopause, sex, the special concerns of lesbian health or a variety of other topics.

Since the first self-help clinic ten years ago, these informal meetings have taken place in homes and offices, on campuses in women's centers and auditoriums, at conventions and conferences, in hotels and dormitories.

When women participate in these groups, they not only learn the means of examining their own anatomy, they also encounter a different way of looking at health care. With an understanding about what is normal for her and how various conditions are related to her overall health, a woman becomes an informed consumer, rather than a passive patient, actively involved in maintaining her health.

The self-help group also offers the opportunity to become acquainted with the extensive body of information which has been reclaimed from the past and gathered by self-helpers through doing vaginal and cervical self-examination in groups, sharing information, operating women's clinics, doing their own research and by researching and writing books.

The self-help clinic is a major foundation of feminist health care. It grew out of the work of laywomen who were concerned with healthy bodily changes rather than disease. Meeting in a supportive, nonjudgmental atmosphere, the self-help clinic breaks down artificial barriers between women imposed upon them by society—barriers which discourage open and unashamed caring about common health concerns, sex or reproduction, and which result in making women who do not fall into the narrow medical definition of "normal" feel unhealthy and unacceptable.

In an introductory session, a woman who is familiar with self-examination starts by talking about the basic concepts of self-help, and, if possible, showing the self-help clinic slide show. She then demonstrates self-examination for the group. After inserting the speculum and taking a look at her own cervix, she offers the other members of the group a look.

Usually women are eager to see their own cervixes after seeing someone else's. If any woman is reluctant to do self-examination in the group, she can take a speculum home with her to look at her cervix for the first time in private.

The reactions of women in a self-help clinic to seeing their cervixes for the first time is varied. Almost all are delighted. Some are amazed. Some are serious. Some are awed by this experience. A typical response is, "You mean it's been there for thirty years and this is the first time I have seen it?"

For many women, being able to *see* the conditions

and changes in their vaginas is a truly revolutionary experience. It gives them a view of their bodies that they never had before. Being able to *see* three or four inches inside the vaginal opening is very different from having what is there described by a doctor from behind a drape, or even having a hurried look through a mirror that a benevolent doctor has handed you.

When doing group self-examination, there are two simple but important courtesies that the group observes. The first is that no woman has to do self-examination if she does not feel comfortable, and the other is that each woman looks at her cervix first, and then, if she wishes, offers the other members a chance to look.

The group can observe the differences in appearance of each other's cervixes. In women who have not had children, the os, or cervical opening, is usually small and round, and in women who have had one or more vaginal deliveries, it tends to be more like a slit. They can observe the variety in color and amount of secretions and each woman can check for warts or pimples on her vulva and cysts or polyps inside the vagina and on the cervix. If anyone has an IUD, they can see where the string comes out and note if secretions have accumulated around it.

Having someone else feel the uterus and possibly the tubes and ovaries, called a uterine size check, is another important part of self-examination. This exam is painful for many women in the doctor's office, but if it is done properly, it should not hurt. Everyone in the group can practice and, with some experience, can learn to identify whether or not a woman has uterine enlargement from pregnancy. After a few sessions of self-help, most women can learn to detect fibroids, growths which sometimes grow either inside or outside of the uterus.

In a self-help clinic, a uterine check is used not to diagnose but to acquaint women with their own anatomy. If anyone notices lumps or swelling in the vaginal area, or tenderness in the pelvic area, she might decide to have her doctor do a uterine check also.

Most women are surprised to learn that Pap smears are very simple to take and that they can do them for each other when they have access to laboratory facilities to have them evaluated.

In addition to acquiring basic self-examination skills, the group then chooses other topics to explore for subsequent meetings. If members are interested in menstrual extraction, they can assemble a Del-Em and discuss the techniques and implications for women's health. Self-helpers can put women who are seriously interested in menstrual extraction in touch with groups who do it on a regular basis.

If the group is interested in discussing sexuality, they can do self-examination of the clitoris and share experiences. Women often find that looking at the clitoris from a feminist perspective takes a lot of mystery out of sex and puts together basic sex information so that it makes sense.

Breast self-examination is a health technique that women often want to learn in a self-help clinic. They are always curious to know why their breasts feel pebbly or lumpy inside and how to distinguish between a cancerous lump and a harmless one. By learning breast self-examination in the group, women can see how healthy breasts differ. They can become less uncomfortable about their own variations.

Groups almost always discuss the menstrual cycle, since it affects every woman for a significant portion of her life! Women who have very long cycles usually think that something is wrong with them and want to know what they can do to "correct" it. Women who have very heavy periods worry that they are losing too much blood and women who have painful cramps are always searching for remedies to ease them. Self-helpers have collected a wealth of information to dispel the myths concerning menstruation and have a store of home remedies for cramps, as well as information on the effects of nutrition and exercise on the menstrual cycle.

Birth control is also a frequent topic in the self-help clinic. Women want to know what effects the Pill has on their bodies, how IUDs work or how to identify their fertile times. Many groups that have access to clinic facilities learn to fit their own diaphragms or cervical caps and to chart their menstrual cycles. Although lesbians or heterosexual women without partners do not need birth control, many have used it in the past and can contribute their experiences. Some have used mucus observation to identify their fertile times in order to become pregnant through donor insemination.

There are so many topics of interest to cover that often an ongoing self-help group develops, perhaps to do menstrual extraction, learn mucus detection and to study the menstrual cycle, or to start a sexuality group. Some specialized self-help groups take up one topic in depth, such as breast cancer, menopause, vaginal infections, herbal remedies or donor insemination.

The self-help clinic is for every woman, whether she is starting to menstruate or has stopped, if she is considering douching, if she is trying to avoid pregnancy or if she is thinking of becoming pregnant, if she has an appointment for a hysterectomy, if she suspects gonorrhea or notices a lump in her breast, if she is having sex with men or with women or not having sex at all. It is a practical, positive approach to health and health care from a feminist point of view.

GLOSSARY

abortion The termination of a pregnancy by any means other than birth.

abstinence In referring to heterosexual women, abstinence means to refrain from having the penis in the vagina. Abstinence does *not* mean refraining from masturbation or other forms of sexual activity.

adrenal gland A triangular-shaped gland attached to the top of each kidney. It secretes various substances that influence every body system. Among the hormones secreted are the steroid hormones: androgens, estrogens and progestogens.

amino acids See *essential amino acids.*

amniotic fluid The transparent liquid contained within the bag of waters (amniotic sac) that surrounds and protects the fetus in the uterus by maintaining even temperature and by providing a cushion from injury.

anal sphincter muscle Part of the doughnut-shaped muscle which surrounds and closes the anus.

androgens A group of steroid hormones which promote the growth and development of muscles, hair and bones.

anteverted The medical term used to describe a uterus that is tipped forward in the pelvis; a normal position.

antibiotic Any natural substance which is used in the treatment of disease to stop or slow the growth of bacteria or other microscopic organisms. Penicillin and tetracycline are two of the most commonly used antibiotics.

antiseptic A substance that prevents decay or hinders the growth of bacteria.

anus The opening at the end of the rectum through which the stool passes.

apocrine glands See *scent glands.*

arginine An amino acid. Eating foods containing arginine—such as cereals, seeds, nuts and chocolates—may promote the growth of herpes.

artificial insemination See *donor insemination.*

astrological computation A method of birth control which works on the principle of determining when a woman will be fertile based on the angular relationship of the sun and moon at the time of her birth. The effectiveness of this method is fairly high because there are relatively few times of the month when unprotected coitus is allowed.

atretic follicle A follicle which never fully developed and shrinks back into the ovary.

"Band-Aid" sterilization See *tubal ligation.*

Bartholin's glands See *vulvovaginal glands.*

basal body temperature The temperature of the body at the time of awakening each morning.

basal body temperature method A way of predicting a woman's fertile time based on observation of the measurable drop and rise in body temperature that commonly occurs around the time of ovulation.

Betadine (povidone-iodine) An iodine-based antibacterial soap that is sold in drug stores without prescription. Betadine makes an effective douche for vaginal bacterial infections or trichomonas.

Billings method A method by which a woman can determine her fertile time by observing cervical mucus on her underpants or toilet paper each day.

biopsy The removal of a small amount of tissue or fluid from the body for diagnostic examination.

bisexual A person who does not exclude the possibility of a sexual relationship with persons of either sex; a term characterizing activity of such a person.

bladder An expandable, muscular sac that holds urine, located behind and above the pubic bone in the lower abdomen.

broad ligament Broad folds of connective tissue attached to the sides of the uterus and extending to the pelvic wall.

bulbocavernosus muscle See *clitoral muscles.*

calendar rhythm A method of estimating a woman's fertile time based on the notion that women ovulate 14 days before their periods. After recording the length of her cycle for about eight months, she calculates her approximate fertile time and abstains from coitus during that period.

Candida albicans See *lactobacillus acidophilus; yeast.*

cannula A strawlike tube which is inserted through the cervical os into the uterus for suctioning its contents. Once made of glass or metal; more modern and safer cannulas are made of flexible plastic.

capillaries The smallest blood vessels in the circulatory system, which form a network throughout the body.

cartilage The part of the skeleton composed of dense, firm tissue which is more flexible than bone. The nose and the pubic symphysis (see page 161) are made of cartilage.

cauterization Destruction of tissue in a localized area by the use of electricity, chemicals, freezing or burning.

cervical canal A narrow passageway, approximately one inch long, within the cervix between the vagina and the uterus. Opening onto the canal are numerous small passageways, which provide a refuge for sperm. Also called the endocervical canal.

cervical cap A barrier method of birth control. The cap, which looks like a large rubber thimble, fits over the cervix and stays on by suction. This method has been used in England and Europe for most of this century.

cervicitis The chronic inflammation or irritation of the cervix.

cervix The lower part of the uterus that extends into the vagina. A woman can usually feel the cervix by putting a finger into her vagina or can see it by using a speculum for self-examination.

chemotherapy Treatment of a disease by chemicals which are usually synthetic. The drugs poison microbes and tissue cells or interfere with their division.

chorionic villi Whitish, branchlike tissue developing in the uterus about two weeks after the union of sperm and egg. This tissue becomes the placenta.

cilia Hairlike structures lining some mucous membranes which move rhythmically to propel secretions and small particles. The cilia that line the egg tubes help move the egg toward the uterus.

clitoral bulbs Two elongated bulbs of spongy erectile tissue lying beneath the outer lips and the bulbocavernosus muscles. They are the equivalent of the single bulb of corpus spongiosum in the penis.

clitoral glans A pea-shaped structure attached to the shaft of the clitoris located beneath the pubic mound. The glans contains a very dense network of blood vessels and for many women is a focal point for sexual stimulation.

clitoral hood A fold of skin that completely covers the clitoral shaft and moves freely over the glans, partially or wholly covering it in an unaroused state.

clitoral legs Extensions of the clitoral shaft that branch out to either side and run alongside the pelvic bone. The legs, also called crura, are made of corpus cavernosum (see below, this page).

clitoral muscles Three sets of muscles that contract during orgasm: the bulbocavernosus muscles, the perineal muscles and the ischiocavernosus muscles.

clitoral shaft A rod of erectile tissue (corpus cavernosum) in the clitoris. Approximately one-half to one inch long, it is bent back on itself and branches out to become the clitoral legs.

clitoris The organ of female orgasm. A complex structure which includes the inner lips, hood, glans, shaft and legs, muscles, urethral sponge, bulbs, networks of nerves and blood vessels, the suspensory ligaments and pelvic diaphragm.

coitus A term which specifically describes sex with the penis in the vagina. It does *not* describe heterosexual sex activities that do not include penis-vagina contact or homosexual sex. This is a nonjudgmental term which does not imply that sex can only take place in the context of a love relationship.

condom A sheath of rubber or animal skin placed on the penis prior to coitus, which catches seminal fluid and prevents sperm from entering the vagina. It also acts as a barrier to bacteria, preventing infections from passing between partners. Condoms are also referred to as sheaths or rubbers.

conization The surgical removal of a cone-shaped core of tissue from the center of the cervix which is then studied for cancerous cells and growths. Also called a cone biopsy.

corpus cavernosum Erectile tissue which fills with blood and becomes bone hard in the plateau phase of sexual response. Seen microscopically, corpus cavernosum consists of bands of involuntary muscles dividing many small hollows or cavities interlaced with capillaries from the clitoral artery. Literally, body of caves.

corpus luteum A small yellow body which develops from the ruptured ovarian follicle after an egg has popped out. It secretes progesterone. If a woman is not pregnant, the corpus luteum shrinks after a few days. If she is pregnant, it keeps on producing hormones.

corpus spongiosum Literally, spongy body. This type of tissue is very similar to the corpus cavernosum except that it contains a more elastic interconnective tissue between the small spaces; therefore, the spongy bodies do not get as hard when erect. The clitoral glans and bulbs are made of corpus spongiosum.

crura See *clitoral legs.*

cryobank A place where frozen tissues are stored until ordered by a doctor or clinic for use. Cryobanks usually have a supply of frozen sperm which can be used for donor insemination.

cryosurgery The destruction of a localized area of tissue by freezing or extreme cold.

crypts The glandular passageways off the cervical canal. Tiny glands at the end of the crypts manufacture mucus which passes out into the cervical canal and into the vagina.

curette A metal instrument, like a cut-out spoon, used to scrape out the uterine contents. The main instrument used in a D and C.

cystic breasts Breasts in which many or frequent cysts or cystic growths occur.

cystitis See *urinary tract infection.*

cysts Pockets or sacs within a tissue or organ usually filled with fluid or semisoft material. Cysts are almost never cancerous.

D and C The opening of the cervical canal for the introduction of a curette in order to scrape the uterine walls. This procedure can be done for the purposes of diagnosis, treatment or abortion.

D and E A method of abortion generally used after the twelfth week of pregnancy, using both suction and tissue forceps to remove the contents of the uterus. Most doctors also use a curette.

Dalkon Shield A plastic, crab-shaped IUD manufactured by the A.H. Robins Company. This IUD has a tendency to become imbedded in the wall of the uterus and causes a high incidence of cervical discharge, irritation and uterine infection. Seventeen deaths were attributed to the Dalkon Shield before it was removed from the market in the United States.

Del-Em A self-help device used to extract the contents of a woman's uterus. It was developed and patented by Lorraine Rothman.

diaphragm A barrier method of birth control which consists of a rubber dome on a flexible rim which covers the cervix and fits behind the pubic bone. The diaphragm requires the use of about a tablespoon of spermicidal cream or jelly. Women who use diaphragms have been found to have fewer vaginal infections, particularly gonorrhea.

dilation The opening of the cervical canal with graduated plastic or metal rods or laminaria so that the instruments used in abortion can enter the uterus. During birth, the cervical canal gradually opens to about ten centimeters, usually by the pressure of the baby's head.

dilation and curettage See *D and C.*

dilation and evacuation See *D and E.*

dilator An instrument used to enlarge or stretch an opening such as the cervical canal.

diuretic A substance which causes an increase in the amount and frequency of urination. Prescription diuretics have numerous ill effects.

donor insemination The introduction of sperm into the vagina or cervical os by some means other than coitus. The procedure is most easily done by using a speculum and inserting sperm into the vagina with a syringe or a turkey baster. Also called artificial insemination. A woman can be assisted in this method of becoming pregnant by a doctor, women in self-help groups or a clinic, or she can do the procedure herself.

douche The introduction of a stream of water or other solution into the vagina. Since the vagina cleanses itself naturally, the main purpose of douching is treatment of vaginal conditions or infections. Although its effectiveness rate is not very high, some women douche as a method of birth control.

dry vagina A condition in which the vagina does not secrete enough mucus to keep it well lubricated or in which the natural secretions have been washed away by douching or in which, prior to coitus, the woman has had insufficient stimulation to lubricate the vagina. Women report itching and pain during coitus from dry vagina. Hormone-like drugs, either taken orally or applied topically, relieve these problems; however, it is not known if a low hormone level is a cause. Exercise, improved nutrition, ointments, adequate stimulation during sex and frequent sex are also effective remedies.

dysmenorrhea Painful menstruation.

dysplasia An unusual development or change in the size, shape or pattern of cells. Some medical professionals think dysplasia is simply a noncancerous growth of a new type of cell.

Early Pregnancy Test (EPT) A two-hour urine pregnancy test which can be purchased at a drug store without a prescription and done at home with the first morning's urine. This test seems to be quite accurate.

egg tubes The tubes or passageways through which the egg travels from the ovary to the uterus. The egg usually unites with the sperm in the lower third of the tube. In medical terminology, they are called fallopian tubes.

embryo The human organism between the second and eighth weeks of development.

endocervical canal See *cervical canal.*

endocrine system Includes thyroid, adrenal glands, pituitary, and ovaries in women and testes in men. These are all ductless glands which secrete hormones and other substances that affect other selected organs of the body directly into the blood stream.

endocrinologists People who study the endocrine system.

endometriosis The condition in which tissue normally found in the uterus is found in other nearby parts of the body. This condition is sometimes accompanied by irregular and painful menstruation or pain during coitus.

engorgement See *vasocongestion.*

episiotomy (clitorotomy) A cut from the vaginal opening into the perineum (see p. 161) to enlarge the vaginal opening during childbirth and to prevent tearing of the perineum. This procedure is not usually necessary, but it is done routinely by most physicians.

erectile tissue A type of tissue found in the clitoris, nipples and penis, made up of many small arteries and cavities, which fills with blood and becomes hard or rigid during sexual response.

erection Erection occurs when sex organs become rigid and elevated as blood fills and becomes trapped in the erectile tissues.

essential amino acids Organic substances which are the "building blocks" of proteins. They are called "essential" because they are necessary for growth and the metabolism of food. They must be obtained from foods, since they cannot be manufactured by the body. Several important protein foods, such as milk, cheese, eggs and meat, contain all of the amino acids considered essential.

estrogens A group of steroid hormones produced in the ovaries and testes and in the adrenal glands of both men and women, and possibly in other tissues, such as body fat. Among their many functions, estrogens are crucial for the healthy growth of skin and mucous membranes. They play a key role in the menstrual cycle by triggering ovulation and by stimulating the growth of the uterine lining.

ethnicity The ethnic group to which a person belongs.

excitement phase The first stage of arousal during sexual excitement.

fallopian tubes See *egg tubes.*

Federation of Feminist Women's Health Centers An organization of women-owned, women-controlled feminist clinics across the United States. Based on self-help, the clinics participate locally and nationally in many feminist health-care projects and issues. The clinics provide well-woman health-care services such as pregnancy screening, general exams, screening and treatment for vaginal infections, birth control, abortion and information on prenatal care and birth.

feedback theory According to this theory, at various points in the menstrual cycle, the rise and fall of blood hormone levels activates the hypothalamus, the pituitary and the ovaries to produce hormones which cause corresponding changes, such as ovulation and menstruation, in the reproductive organs.

feminist A person who favors and works for women's rights. A radical feminist believes that the oppression of women is a result of a patriarchal system and recognizes the necessary connection between women achieving equality and the rights of all oppressed classes, ethnic groups and minority groups.

fertile mucus Mucus secretion from the cervix which generally occurs around the time of ovulation. It is alkaline and stretchy like egg whites. Fertile mucus helps propel sperm into the uterus.

fertile period The time in a woman's menstrual cycle when an egg is likely to be fertilized if sperm enter the uterus and egg tubes.

fetus A developing human from three months to birth.

fibroids Fibrous, noncancerous growths, most commonly found in or on the uterus.

follicle A small, round sac. In the ovary, each egg is contained in a follicle.

follicle-stimulating hormone (FSH) A hormone secreted by the pituitary gland. It is thought that when the level of this hormone rises in the bloodstream after menstruation, it stimulates a number of follicles in the ovary to grow and mature.

frenulum The part of the clitoris where the underside of the glans and inner lips meet.

front commisure The area just above the clitoral shaft on the pubic mound.

fundus The top part of the uterus.

general anesthetic Any drug that blocks sensations in the body by producing paralysis or unconsciousness. Bodily processes such as breathing, heartbeat, blood pressure and bowel activity are slowed down.

genital warts Small, rough bumps on, in or near the genitals caused by a virus. Warts are generally painless, but can cause irritation to the tissues nearby. They can bleed if scratched or irritated. Also called venereal warts.

genitals The organs of sexual pleasure and reproduction which, in women, include the clitoris, vulva, vagina, uterus, urethra, egg tubes and ovaries. In men, they include the testes, their excretory ducts, the penis, urethra and prostate gland.

gonorrhea A sexually transmitted disease caused by the bacterium *Neisseria gonorrhoeae*. It is transmitted by a person carrying the bacteria when one mucous membrane comes in contact with another, or when any warm, moist part of the body comes together with another. If not treated, this disease can cause severe infection and sterility. Also called VD (venereal disease) or "the clap."

herpes A viral disease that causes the skin to erupt in recurring blisters, most commonly on the genitals and mouth. Herpes can be spread when herpes blisters come in contact with mucous membranes, an open sore or a cut.

heterosexual A term referring to sexual activity between a woman and a man, or to a person who chooses to relate sexually to the opposite sex.

homosexual A term referring to sexual activity between persons of the same sex, or to a person who chooses to relate sexually to the same sex.

hormones Minute substances manufactured in organs, glands or tissues which are transported in the bloodstream to distant parts of the body to stimulate specific activity or production of other hormones. These naturally occurring chemicals affect every part of the body and are directly affected by environmental influences such as nutrition, exercise, stress, temperature and light.

hot flashes A feeling of heat in the body lasting a few seconds to several minutes. Sometimes the face becomes red or flushed and sweating occurs. Some people feel chilled afterward. No one knows what causes hot flashes, but they have been linked to hormonal changes.

hymen A membrane approximately one inch within the clitoral opening to the vagina. The size, shape, thickness and the degree to which it closes off the vaginal opening vary from woman to woman. The hymen also varies in appearance at different times during a woman's life.

hypoglycemia Low blood sugar. The point at which an insufficient amount of sugar (glucose) is present in the bloodstream. Some symptoms of hypoglycemia are cold sweats, goose bumps, irritability, trembling or shaking, lowered body temperature, extreme fatigue and, in more serious cases, chronic fainting, coma or convulsions.

hysterectomy The surgical removal of the uterus. A radical hysterectomy includes removal of the uterus, cervix, vaginal tissue next to the cervix, the egg tubes, ovaries and sometimes the lymph nodes nearby.

informed consent Ensuring that a patient has full information about examinations, tests, procedures or drugs before treatment is given, including possible risks and complications of any kind and whether a drug or treatment is experimental.

inner lips of the clitoris Two parallel folds of skin surrounding the urethra and the clitoral opening to the vagina. Part of the clitoris, the inner lips swell and undergo dramatic color changes during sexual excitement. Also called small lips or *labia minora*.

inverted nipple A nipple whose tip sinks in instead of standing out. This condition is not a health problem, and women who want to breast-feed can correct the shape of the nipple by repeatedly drawing it out with the fingers, or they can let the baby's sucking bring it out.

involuntary muscles Certain muscles which contract automatically rather than by conscious effort.

ischiocavernosus muscle A muscle which runs along the legs of the clitoris and which contracts during sexual response.

IUD (intrauterine device) Commercial IUDs are short plastic rods bent into different shapes and sometimes wound with copper wire and inserted into the uterus for the purpose of birth control. Although it is not clear how the IUD works, it usually prevents a fertilized egg from implanting on the uterine wall.

Lactobacillus acidophilus A class of "friendly" bacteria found in yogurt and other milk products. It is also found in both the intestines and the vagina, where it keeps the growth of yeast down. When *Lactobacillus acidophilus* is introduced into the vagina in the form of plain yogurt, tablets or a douche, it can decrease yeast overgrowth.

Laetrile therapy A controversial anticancer treatment in which a form of amygdalin (also called vitamin B-17), a compound extracted from foods such as almonds and apricot seeds, is taken along with other nutritional therapy.

laminaria Compressed sticks of sterile, dried seaweed, about the size of kitchen matches, which are inserted through the os into the cervical canal. Cervical secretions moisten the seaweed which causes it to slowly expand and stretch the cervical os and canal. Some laminaria expand in about six hours and some expand over a longer time, up to 12 hours, or overnight.

laparoscopy Examination of the interior of the abdomen by means of a laparoscope; also the closing of the egg tubes by burning them shut (electrocautery) with a laparoscope which has been inserted through an incision beneath the navel.

laparotomy Any surgery done through an abdominal incision.

lesbian There are many political and social aspects of lesbianism, but for the purposes of health, a lesbian is a woman who prefers to have sexual relationships only with women.

libido A Freudian term that has come to mean sexual desire or sex drive.

local anesthetic An application of pain-killer to the part of the body where a procedure is to be done. For an abortion, it is an injection given directly into the cervix.

lumpectomy The surgical removal of a breast tumor and sometimes other breast tissue without removing the entire breast.

luteinizing hormone (LH) A hormone manufactured in the pituitary gland which is believed to stimulate the ovary to secrete steroid hormones and to stimulate the formation of the corpus luteum (yellow body), a glandular structure which forms from the ruptured follicle after ovulation.

lymph nodes Enclosed masses of tissue that vary from the size of a tiny dot to the size of a marble. Lymph nodes filter out foreign particles, such as bacteria, preventing them from entering the bloodstream.

lysine an essential amino acid found in dairy products, meat, potatoes, yeast and other foods. (These foods also contain arginine in smaller quantities.) Some research has suggested that a high intake of lysine may help suppress or shorten the duration of an outbreak of herpes.

mammography A controversial method of photographing the breast by using X-rays. The procedure is intended to reveal or confirm breast lumps. The routine use of mammography is now only recommended for women who have a high risk of developing breast cancer.

mastectomy The surgical removal of breast tissue, which ranges from removal of a small part of the breast to removal of the entire breast, lymph nodes, fat, muscles and surrounding skin.

masturbation Physical or mental stimulation of one's own body, particularly the genitals, to produce sexual pleasure and orgasm.

menopause The time in a woman's life—usually in her forties or fifties—during which the menstrual pattern changes, ultimately resulting in a cessation of the menstrual activity. It is easier to judge retrospectively when menopause has occurred.

menstrual extraction Removal of the uterine contents by suction on or about the first day of the menstrual period, done by women in self-help groups with a Del-Em.

metabolism The sum of chemical changes, the building up or destruction of cells, which take place in the body.

Mittelschmerz Literally, middle pain. A sharp pain often felt low in the abdomen on one side or the other which is thought to be caused by ovulation.

Monilia See *yeast.*

mucous membrane A thin layer of tissue lining the body cavities that come into direct or indirect contact with the outside. Mucous membranes are kept moist by the secretions of mucus-producing glands.

nonfertile mucus The type of cervical mucus that is present for most of a woman's cycle, except around the time she is ovulating. This mucus has a watery or slightly pasty quality, is acidic and appears under a microscope to have a tightly woven structure which prevents the passage of sperm into the cervical canal.

nonspecific vaginitis A medical term for a bacterial infection of the vagina. It is "nonspecific" when several different types of bacteria may be present or when the type of bacteria is not known.

orgasm The culmination of sexual tension in muscle contractions which force out accumulated blood from erect and engorged genital tissues.

orgasmic platform A phrase used by Masters and Johnson to support their mistaken belief that orgasms originate in the vagina. They classify structures such as the clitoral bulbs, urethral sponge, inner lips, perineal sponge and blood vessels as "the outer third of the vagina" or "orgasmic platform."

os The mouth of the uterus. The opening at either end of the cervical canal. The opening into the uterus is the inner os; the opening into the vagina is the outer os.

outer lips of the clitoris Two fatty, protective folds outside the inner lips that are parallel and extend from the pubic mound to the perineum. Also called large lips or *labia majora.*

ovaries Two white endocrine glands about the size of unshelled almonds, located on either side of the pelvic cavity near the opening of the egg tubes. From birth through old age, they produce hormones—estrogens, progestogens and androgens. During a woman's reproductive years, they release ripe eggs.

ovulation The point in a woman's menstrual cycle when an egg ripens and breaks through the wall of the ovary.

Pap smear A screening for cancer of the cervix. Samples of cells from the face of the cervix, the os and the vagina are smeared on a slide for examination to determine whether they have any unusual characteristics which might indicate cancer.

papillomas Harmless, wartlike growths generally located on the skin or mucous membranes. Papillomas can grow on any part of the body and are occasionally found on the breast.

paraurethral ducts and glands Two very small ducts and glands just inside the urethra. Their function is not known. A woman is never aware of them unless they become infected. They are believed to be the source of secretion in female ejaculation.

patient advocate Someone who accompanies a person through an examination or medical procedure to give emotional support and to try to ensure that the person is treated respectfully, that questions are answered and that all necessary tests are done. The advocate also helps to ensure that the person being examined has complete information about which procedures are being done, the reasons for doing them and the options of requesting or refusing any drugs or procedures.

pectoral muscles Muscles attached to the upper part of the chest.

pelvic diaphragm The muscular floor of the pelvis, formed by the pubococcygeal muscle and a second large muscle. These two muscles separate the pelvis from the perineum.

penis The male organ of orgasm, reproduction and urination. A complex structure which includes glans, foreskin, bulbocavernosus muscle, corpus spongiosum, urogenital diaphragm, bulbourethral gland, legs (crura), suspensory ligament and a complex network of nerves and blood vessels. *Note:* Despite the differences in size and arrangement, the components of the clitoris and the penis are nearly the same.

perineal muscles See *clitoral muscles.*

perineal sponge An area of spongy erectile tissue and blood vessels beneath the perineum, which fills with blood during sexual response.

perineum The bridge of flesh between the vaginal opening and the anus. This area is cut, often unnecessarily, during childbirth.

pituitary gland A kidney-bean-sized endocrine gland located at the base of the brain which is responsible for the production of a wide variety of hormones—particularly follicle-stimulating hormone (FSH) and luteinizing hormone (LH)—which appear to be responsible for stimulating the formation of the corpus luteum after ovulation and the secretion of steroid hormones in both the ovaries and testes.

placenta The oval-shaped spongy structure that is formed in early pregnancy to filter nutrients to the fetus while filtering out waste products. The placenta is attached to the uterine wall and the fetus is attached to the placenta by the umbilical cord.

plateau phase The phase of sexual response, marked by intense sexual excitement, just prior to orgasm.

polyps Soft red growths with stems that most commonly occur in organs such as the uterus and rectum, which have a rich supply of blood. Polyps are usually noncancerous, but can cause a discharge or can bleed when irritated.

population control The attempt of the state to determine the birth rate, death rate, and migration or mobility within the society by regulation, custom and behavior. Population control is often influenced or carried out by government policies, legal decisions, economic incentives, medical policies, religious institutions, private foundations and the media.

precancerous A term describing a condition which has the potential for becoming cancerous later. Most so-called precancerous conditions do *not* become cancer, but watching for changes and frequent testing are important.

primary follicle An ovarian follicle or sac which is composed of a single layer of cells surrounding the egg. Until stimulated to grow and develop, all ovarian follicles are at a primary stage.

progesterone A steroid hormone manufactured in the corpus luteum and adrenal glands which promotes the growth of the uterine lining prior to menstruation and, in pregnancy, the growth of the placenta.

progestogens A group of steroid hormones which include progesterone and other hormones which have similar effects.

proliferative phase One of the three phases of the menstrual cycle. After menstruation, the uterine lining becomes thicker with an increased blood supply. During this phase, the maturing ovarian follicle secretes estrogens. This phase usually lasts from 10 to 13 days.

pubic bone The lower front part of the pelvic bone.

pubic symphysis The area where the pelvic bones meet underneath the pubic mound.

pubococcygeal muscle A broad band of muscles that forms a sling from the pubic bone to the tail bone. This muscle surrounds the vagina, urethra and rectum and can be voluntarily contracted. The muscle also contracts involuntarily during orgasm.

pyridium A drug used to suppress symptoms and prevent discomfort in severe urinary tract infections. Pyridium does not kill bacteria, but is often prescribed along with antibiotics for UTI.

racism Bias or prejudice that results in discrimination or oppression based on a person's (usually a person of color) race.

rad Radiation-absorbed dose. A defined unit of absorbed energy used to determined the amount of X-ray dosage a person should be given.

radiation therapy The treatment of cancer with radioactive elements to destroy cancerous cells.

rectovaginal exam An examination of the uterus, egg tubes and ovaries which is done by inserting the gloved middle finger into the rectum and the index finger into the vagina, while the other hand is used to press down on the abdomen. This exam is done if the uterus is difficult to feel vaginally.

rectum The lower part of the large intestine that extends to the anus.

resolution phase The phase of sexual response after orgasm when the body returns to an unexcited state.

retroverted The medical term used to describe a uterus which is tipped backward in the body toward the tail bone. A perfectly normal position.

round ligament A cordlike ligament attached to the uterus in front of the egg tubes. It extends to the outer lips.

saline abortion An induced miscarriage in which a small amount of amniotic fluid is withdrawn from the uterus through a hollow needle and three to four cups of sterile saline solution (salt water) are replaced. The salt water kills the fetus and stimulates the uterus to contract to expel it.

scent glands The glands which secrete under conditions of excitement, stress, pain or fear. They are called the "scent" glands since their fluid is the key ingredient needed for the formation of human odor. They are located predominantly in the armpits, pubic and anal areas. The milk glands are also of this type. These glands are also called the apocrine glands.

secondary follicle A follicle which has partly developed and has several layers of cells which secrete a jellylike fluid around the egg.

secretory phase The phase of the menstrual cycle immediately after ovulation. The uterine lining increases in thickness; its glands become more twisted and secrete an abundant mucus containing glycogen. The uterine lining becomes puffy with water. The corpus luteum is active. This phase usually lasts between 10 and 14 days.

seminal fluid The thick, white secretion produced by a man's reproductive organs which passes through the urethra of the penis during orgasm. The seminal fluid contains the sperm, as well as secretions from various glands.

sexism Bias or prejudice that results in the descrimination or oppression based on a person's (usually a woman's) sex.

shaft of the clitoris The shaft, a round rubbery-feeling cord made of corpus cavernosum, connects the glans of the clitoris to its legs. It is highly sensitive and moves when touched.

speculum An instrument, usually metal or plastic, which is inserted into a body opening in order to look at the cavity wall and its contents. Vaginal speculums are used to see the vagina and cervix.

sperm Microscopic tadpole-shaped cells produced in a man's body, which are passed out through the urethra in the seminal fluid. When a sperm is united with an egg, it develops within the uterus first into an embryo and then into a fetus.

spermicidal cream or jelly A cream or jelly that kills sperm. In actual use, a spermicide will kill *most* of the sperm in the vagina.

squamocolumnar junction The rim where the lining of the cervical canal (made up of column-shaped cells) meets the flat cells of the face of the cervix. If the column-shaped squamous cells grow outside of the cervical canal, they form a visible red circle around the os.

sterilization abuse Sterilization in any form including hysterectomy imposed on people, usually women of color, poor women or older women, without their full informed consent or knowledge.

steroid hormones A class of hormones formed from cholesterol, namely, estrogens, progestogens and androgens, as well as a group of hormones secreted by the adrenal glands.

stirrups Two footrests that are positioned at the end of an exam table during most pelvic exams, childbirth and surgery. It is not medically necessary for a woman to use stirrups during most procedures if she does not want to.

superficial cells The top layer of cells of the vaginal lining. Under hormonal influence, the cells of the vaginal lining increase rapidly; as new cells grow from the base of the lining, they push older cells upward to the surface. These cells become flattened and, as they reach the top, they die and are sloughed off. These older cells are termed superficial.

surgery The branch of medicine which deals with injury, disease or structural changes by using procedures that cut into the body for diagnosis or treatment.

suspensory ligament A ligament that attaches the shaft of the clitoris or penis to the pubic symphysis.

tertiary follicle At some point prior to ovulation, the secondary follicles inside the ovary begin to shrink, leaving one which continues to grow to as much as half the size of the ovary. This follicle, or sac, contains an egg and is called a tertiary follicle, signifying the third stage of growth.

thermography A method of detecting the presence of cysts by measuring temperature differences among tissues. Cysts grow faster than the surrounding tissue and therefore give off more heat, which can be detected by this method.

transillumination A method used in confirming the presence and size of breast lumps by shining a very strong light through the breast.

trichomonas An infection caused by microscopic, single-celled parasites which live in the vaginal tissue, *Trichomonas vaginalis.* Typically the major symptom is a greenish or yellowish discharge with a strong, unpleasant odor, which has been variously described as "fishy," "acrid" or "swampy."

tubal ligation Surgically blocking the egg tubes to prevent the union of sperm and egg.

urethral sponge A sheath of corpus spongiosum erectile tissue around the urethra which becomes engorged during sexual excitement and protects the urethra during sexual activity.

urinary tract infection (UTI) An inflammation or infection in the bladder which can sometimes spread to the kidneys. The cause can be stress, sexual activity or improper wiping after a bowel movement. The location of the urethra makes some women more prone to frequent infections. The infection can be caused by a number of different kinds of bacteria.

urine pregnancy test A test used to determine the presence of the pregnancy hormone in the urine. The test is accurate for most women about 41 days from the first day of the last normal menstrual period, or about two weeks after a period has been missed.

urogenital diaphragm The muscles that form a platform for the clitoris. The vagina and the urethra pass through it.

uterine size check An examination in which two fingers of one hand are inserted into the vagina to touch the cervix, and the abdomen is pressed just above the pubic hairline with the other hand. The objective is to feel the normal size and position of the uterus. The egg tubes and ovaries can be checked at the same time.

uterine ligaments See *round ligament, broad ligament* and *suspensory ligament.*

uterus A muscular, hollow, pear-shaped organ with an inner mucous membrane lining, the endometrium. It lies in the middle of the pelvis, supported by several ligaments. Its three parts are the cervix, the main body and the fundus. The uterus undergoes changes in the sexual response cycle; the endometrium goes through monthly cyclic changes throughout a woman's life; and during pregnancy, the uterus houses the fetus.

vagina The very elastic canal with a mucous membrane lining which extends from the cervix to the vulva. The vaginal walls usually touch each other, but can be greatly expanded, especially during childbirth. Also called the birth canal.

vasocongestion The filling of tissue by blood during the sexual response cycle, causing swelling of the veins and closing of the valves. Vasocongestion traps blood in the tissues and causes swelling of the breasts and sex organs and reddening or duskiness of the surface skin.

venereal disease (VD) Sexually transmitted diseases which include syphilis, gonorrhea, herpes and trichomonas.

venereal warts See *genital warts.*

venous lakes Pockets in the uterine lining where blood accumulates just before menstruation begins. These pockets burst, contributing blood and dead cells to the menstrual flow.

vulvovaginal glands A pair of mucus-secreting glands approximately the size and shape of a lima bean with openings at the lower part of the inner lips.

white body An old corpus luteum which shrinks back into the ovary.

Women's Health Movement The Women's Health Movement is composed of individuals and groups who are working to improve women's and infants' health care, women's reproductive and sexual freedom and the status and power of women health workers, both paid and unpaid. Issues of special interest are: occupational health, abortion, sterilization abuse, childbirth, unsafe birth control, excessive surgery, lack of informed consent, substance abuse, patient advocacy, home health workers, lay health workers, rape and other forms of violence against women, aging, and status of nurses. Self-help is an approach to the solution of these and other problems and is based on the idea that women have been controlled through the suppression of their sexuality, and the belief that if women can learn directly about their bodies through self-examination together, they can regain sexual and reproductive control.

xeroradiography A photoelectric method of X-raying a woman's breasts to detect cysts or tumors.

yeast A fungus normally present in the vagina and rectum which can overgrow and cause discomfort. Also called *Monilia* or *Candida albicans.*

yogurt A fermented, semisolid milk product which has become a standard home remedy for yeast conditions in the vagina. Plain, unpasteurized yogurt containing *Lactobacillus acidophilus* or *Lactobacillus bulgaricus* is the most effective kind to use.

APPENDIX: WOMEN'S HEALTH PROJECTS

The following is a list of Feminist health care facilities which provide abortions and a list of feminist health clinics and projects. Feminist, women-controlled clinics which provide abortion are indicated by +. Feminist health clinics and projects which do not do abortions, but do make referrals are indicated by *.

Arkansas

* Mari Spehar Health Education Project
  Box 545
  Fayetteville, Arkansas 72701

California

* Bay Area Healing Tao
  P.O. Box 460195
  San Francisco, California 94146
  (415) 731-1166

* Berkeley Women's Health Collective
  2908 Ellsworth
  Berkeley, California 94705
  (510) 843-6194

+ Chico Feminist Women's Health Center
  1469 Humboldt Road, Number 200
  Chico, California 95928
  (916) 891-1911

* Committee to Defend Reproductive Rights
  558 Capp Street
  San Francisco, California 94110
  (415) 647-2694

* DES Action
  1615 Broadway, Number 510
  Oakland, California 94612
  (510) 465-4011

* Federation of Feminist Women's Health Centers
  633 East 11th Avenue
  Eugene, Oregon 97401
  (503) 344-0966

* Gentle Birth Center
  1989 Riverside Drive
  Los Angeles, California 90039
  (818) 545-7128

* Lesbian Health Project
  Lesbian Health Clinic &
  Donor Insemination Program
  8240 Santa Monica Boulevard
  Los Angeles, California 90046
  (213) 650-1508

* Lyon Martin Women's Health Services
  1784 Market Street, Suite 201
  San Francisco, California 94102
  (415) 565-7667

* North Country Clinic for Women and Children
  785 - 18th Street
  Arcata, California 95521
  (707) 822-2481

+ Redding Feminist Women's Health Center
  1901 Victor Avenue
  Redding, California 96002
  (916) 221-0193

+ Sacramento Feminist Women's Health Center
  3401 Folsom Boulevard, Suite A
  Sacramento, California 95816
  (916) 451-0621

* Santa Cruz Women's Health Collective
  250 Locust Street
  Santa Cruz, California 95060
  (408) 427-3500

* Sperm Bank of California
  Reproductive Technologies
  2115 Milvia, 2nd Floor
  Berkeley, California 94704
  (510) 841-1858

+ Westside Women's Health Center
  1711 Ocean Park Boulevard
  Santa Monica, California 90405
  (310) 450-2191

* Wholistic Health For Women
  8240 Santa Monica Boulevard
  Los Angeles, California 90046
  (213) 650-1508

+ Womancare, A Feminist Women's Health Center
  2850 - 6th Avenue, Suite 311
  San Diego, California 92103
  (619) 298-9352

+ Womancare - South
  688 Hollister Street, Apt. B
  San Diego, California 92154
  (619) 424-9944

Connecticut
*Women's Health Services
  911 State Street
  New Haven, Connecticut 06511
  (203) 777-4781

Florida
+ Feminist Women's Health Center
  241 East 6th Avenue
  Tallahassee, Florida 32303
  (904) 224-9600

+ Gainesville Women's Health Center
  720 North West 23rd Avenue
  Gainesville, Florida 32609
  (904) 377-5055

Georgia
+ Feminist Women's Health Center
  580 14th Street, North West
  Atlanta, Georgia 30318
  (404) 874-7551

Illinois
* Chicago Women's Health Center
  3435 North Sheffield
  Chicago, Illinois
  (312) 935-6126

Iowa
+ Cedar Rapids Clinic for Women
  4089 - 21st Avenue South West
  Cedar Rapids, Iowa 52404
  (319) 390-4342

+Emma Goldman Clinic for Women
  227 North Dubuque
  Iowa City, Iowa 52245
  (319) 337-2111

Maine
+ Mabel Wadsworth Women's Health Center
  334 Harlow
  Bangor, Maine 94401
  (207) 947-5337

Massachusetts
* Boston Women's Health Book Collective
  240 "A" Elm Avenue
  Summerville, Massachusetts 02144
  (617) 625-0271

* Everywoman's Center Health Project
  University of Massachusetts
  Wilder Hall
  Amherst, Massachusetts 01003
  (413) 545-0883

* New Bedford Women's Center
  252 County Street
  New Bedford, Massachusetts 02740
  (508) 996-3343

Missouri
* Women's Self-Help Center
  2838 Olive Street
  St. Louis Missouri 63103
  (314) 531-2003

Montana

+ Blue Mountain Women's Clinic
610 California
Missoula, Montana 59802
(406) 721-1646

New Hampshire

+ Feminist Health Center
38 South Main Street
Concord, New Hampshire 03301
(603) 225-2739

+ Portsmouth Feminist Health Center
PO Box 45
Greenland, New Hampshire 03840
(603) 436-7588

New Mexico

* Women's Health Services
141 Paseo De Peralta
Santa Fe, New Mexico 87501
(505) 988-8869

New York

* Community Health Project
Lesbian Health Program
208 West 13th Street
New York, New York 10011
(212) 675-3559

* Womancap
25 - 5th Avenue
New York, New York 10003
(212) 529-8498

Oregon

+ Eugene Feminist Women's Health Center
633 East 11th
Eugene, Oregon 97401
(541) 342-5940

+ Portland Feminist Women's Health Center
1020 North East 2nd, Suite 200
Portland, Oregon 97232
(503) 233-0808

Pennsylvania

+ Elizabeth Blackwell Health Center for Women
1124 Walnut Street, 2nd Floor
Philadelphia, Pennsylvania 19107
(215) 923-1124

Rhode Island

* Rhode Island Women's Health Collective
500 Prospect
Pawtucket, Rhode Island 02860
(401) 726-7477

Vermont

+ Southern Vermont Women's Health Center
187 North Main Street
Rutland, Vermont 05701
(802) 775-1946

+ Vermont Women's Health Center
336 North Avenue
Burlington, Vermont 05401
(802) 863-1386

Washington

+ Aradia Women's Health Center
1300 Spring Street
Seattle, Washington 98122
(206) 323-9388

+ Cedar River Clinic
4300 Talbot Road South
Renton, Washington 98655
(206) 255-0471

+ Yakima Feminist Women's Health Center
106 East "E" Street
Yakima, Washington 98901
(509) 575-6422

Washington, D.C.

* National Black Women's Health Project
1211 Connecticut North West, Number 310
Washington, D.C. 20036
(202) 835-0117

* National Women's Health Network
514 10th Street North West, Number 400
Washington, D.C. 20004
(202) 347-1140

West Virginia

+ Women's Health Center of West Virgina
3418 Staunton Avenue, South East
Charleston, West Virgina 25304
(304) 344-9834

Canada

+ Every Woman's Health Clinic
  2005 East 44th Avenue
  Vancouver, British Columbia V5P 1N1
  Canada
  (604) 322-6692

* Vancouver Women's Health Collective
  Number 219 - 1675 West 8th Avenue
  Vancouver, British Columbia V6J 1V2
  Canada
  (604) 736-5262

Mexico

* Tijuana Self-Help Clinic
  C/O Zelina Espinoza
  Calle Pico Pico Numero 1442 Altos 5-A
  La Mesa, Tijuana, Baja California
  Mexico
  011-5266-826024

BIBLIOGRAPHY

Anonymous, Sarah and Mary. *Woman Controlled Conception.* San Francisco: Womanshare Books, 1979. (Available from Gay Teachers and School Workers, 3939 24th Street, San Francisco, CA 94114. *$2.)*

The Boston Women's Health Book Collective. *Our Bodies, Ourselves.* Revised and expanded. New York: Simon and Schuster, 1979.

Cherniak, Donna. *A Book About Birth Control.* Montreal: The Montreal Health Press, 1979.

Cherniak, Donna, and Allan Feingold. *VD Handbook.* Montreal: The Montreal Health Press, 1977.

Corea, Gena. *The Hidden Malpractice: How American Medicine Mistreats Women.* New York: William Morrow and Company, Inc. 1977; New York: Jove, 1978.

Cowan, Belita. *Women's Health Care: Resources, Writings, Bibliographies.* Ann Arbor: Anshen Publishing Co., 1977. (Also available from the author: 3821 T Street, N.W., Washington, D.C., 20007. *$3.)*

Delaney, Janice, Mary Jane Lupton and Emily Toth. *The Curse.* New York: New American Library, 1977.

Downer, Carol. "Self-Help for Sex." *Women's Sexual Development,* edited by Martha Kirkpatrick, M.D. New York: Plenum Publishing Corporation, 1980.

Ehrenreich, Barbara, and John Ehrenreich. *The American Health Empire.* New York: Random House, 1970.

Ehrenreich, Barbara, and Dierdre English. *Witches, Midwives and Nurses: A History of Women Healers.* Glass Mountain Pamphlets. (Available from The Feminist Press, Box 334, Old Westbury, NY 11568.)

Ehrenreich, Barbara, and Dierdre English. *For Her Own Good.* New York: Doubleday/Anchor Books, 1978.

Gage, Suzann. *When Birth Control Fails . . . How to Abort Ourselves Safely.* Los Angeles: Speculum Press, 1979. (Available from Speculum Press, PO Box 1063, Los Angeles, CA 90028.)

Graedon, Joe. *The People's Pharmacy: A Guide to Prescription Drugs, Home Remedies and Over the Counter Medications.* New York: St. Martin's Press, 1976.

Hatcher, Robert, M.D., et al. *Contraceptive Technology.* 10th Edition, New York: Irvington Publishers, Inc., 1980.

Hite, Shere. *The Hite Report.* New York: Dell Publishing Company, 1976.

Hornstein, Francie. *Lesbian Health Care.* 1974. (Available from the Feminist Women's Health Center, 6411 Hollywood Boulevard, Los Angeles, CA 90028.)

Kilmartin, Angela. *Understanding Cystitis.* London: Heineman Health Books, 1973.

Kittler, Glenn D. *Laetrile: Nutritional Control for Cancer with Vitamin B-17.* Denver: Royal Publications, Inc., 1978.

Kushner, Rose. *If You've Thought About Breast Cancer.* Washington, D.C.: Office of Cancer Communications, National Cancer Institute. (Also available from the National Women's Health Network, 224 7th Street, S.E., Washington, D.C. 20003 at no cost.)

Kushner, Rose. *Why Me? What Every Woman Should Know About Breast Cancer to Save Her Life.* New York: Signet, 1977.

Lappe, Frances Moore, and Joseph Collins. *Food First.* Boston: Houghton Mifflin Co., 1977.

Lader, Lawrence. *Abortion II: Making the Revolution.* Boston: Beacon Press, 1973.

Levin, Arthur. "Mammography: A Case for Informed Consent." (Available from Health Research Group, Department P, 2000 P Street, N.W., Washington, D.C. 20036.)

Morgan, Robin. *Sisterhood is Powerful.* New York: Vintage Books, 1970.

Morgan, Suzanne. *Hysterectomy.* 1978. (Available from the author, 2921 Walnut Avenue, Manhattan Beach, CA 90266. Also from the National Women's Health Network, 224 7th Street, S.E., Washington, D.C. 20003.)

National Women's Health Network Guides on (1) *Breast Cancer;* (2) *Hysterectomy;* (3) *Menopause;* (4) *Maternal Health and Childbirth;* (5) *Birth Control;* (6) *DES:* (7) *Self-Help;* (8) *Abortion.* Available from National Women's Health Network, 224 7th Street, S.E., Washington, D.C. 20003.

Nelson, Chris. *Self-Help Home Remedies.* 1977. (Available from Chico Feminist Women's Health Center, 330 Flume Street, Chico, CA 95926, **$2.**)

O'Donnell, Mary. "Lesbian Health Care: Issues and Literature." *Science for the People* (May/June, 1978), pages 8–19.

Punnett, Laura. "Menstrual Extraction: Politics." **Quest 4** 3 (Summer, 1978). (Available from the Feminist Women's Health Center, 6411 Hollywood Boulevard, Los Angeles, CA 90028.)

Reitz, Rosetta. *Menopause: A Positive Approach.* Radnor, Pa.: Chilton Books, 1977; New York: Penguin, 1979.

Rothman, Lorraine. "Menstrual Extraction: Procedures." *Quest 4* 3 (Summer, 1978). (Available from the Feminist Women's Health Center, 6411 Hollywood Boulevard, Los Angeles, CA 90028.)

Ruzek, Sheryl. *The Women's Health Movement: Feminist Alternatives to Medical Control.* New York: Praeger Special Studies, 1978.

Santa Cruz Women's Health Collective. "Herpes." (1978). (Available from the authors, 250 Locust Street, Santa Cruz, CA 95060, $1.50).

Santa Cruz Women's Health Collective. Lesbian Health Matters (1977). (Available from the authors, 250 Locust Street, Santa Cruz, CA 95060, $4).

Seaman, Barbara, and Gideon Seaman, M.D. *Women and the Crisis in Sex Hormones.* New York: Rawson Associates Publishers, Inc., 1977; New York: Bantam Books, 1978.

Seaman, Barbara. *The Doctor's Case Against the Pill.* New York: Peter Wyden, 1969; New York: Dell, 1979.

Sherfey, Mary Jane, M.D. *The Nature and Evolution of Female Sexuality.* New York: Vintage Books, 1973.

Stone, Irwin. *The Healing Factor: Vitamin C Against Disease.* New York: Grosset and Dunlap, 1972.

Weiss, Kay. "Cancer and Estrogens: A Review." *Women and Health* 1:2 (March/April, 1976).

INDEX

abortion, 129-35
  aspiration, 121, 129, 130, 132-33, 146
  complications of, 130, 131
  D and C, 145, 146
  D and E, 130, 131
  early-termination, 121, 129
  illegal, 131
  incomplete, 131
  menstrual extraction, 121-27
  nontraumatic, 18, 19, 129-30, 135
  organizing in support of, 18
  referrals for, 18
  saline, 131, 135
  sites for, 130-31
abortion clinics, women-controlled, 19,
  129-31
abstinence, 108, 119
Abzug, Bella, 19
Achilles tendon, relaxation technique and,
  100
acidic liquids, 101
adrenal glands, hormones produced by, 66,
  70
aging, 76
aloe vera gel, 76, 91
American Psychological Association, 19
American Public Health Association, 19
androgens, 70
  functions of, 66
anesthesia:
  abortion and, 129, 130, 131, 145
  surgery and, 137-38, 141, 144, 145
antibiotics, 89, 101, 131
anus, 37, 38, 40
appetite, changes in, 83
arginine, 90
arm pain, 109
armpits, lymph nodes in, 29
artificial insemination, 85
astrological computation, birth control and,
  106, 120

back pain, relief of, 98

baking soda, 102, 115
"Band Aid" surgery, 144-45
Bartholin's glands, *see* vulvovaginal glands
basal body temperature, 106-7, 119
Betadine douche, 89, 93
Billings method, 119, 120
biopsies, 137, 139, 150
birth control, 104-20
  bias in choice of, 105
  effectiveness of, 105, 115, 119-20
  safety factors and, 19, 105-6, 108-9, 118
  see also specific methods
birth control pills, *see* Pill, the
black women, 145
bladder, 35, 50, 65, 97, 147
  see also urinary tract infections
bleeding:
  abortion and, 131
  drug-withdrawal, 105-6
  fibroids and, 97
  IUDs and, 117
  menstrual extraction and, 127
  polyps and, 95
  during urination, 100, 101
  see also menstruation, menstrual cycle
blood clots, 109
blood pressure, 50, 102
BME (Board of Medical Examiners,
  California), 18
bones, brittleness of, 76
bow exercise, 99
breastfeeding, 69, 141
breasts:
  cancer of, 109, 138-43
  cystic, 30, 31, 86, 87, 138, 140
  differences in size of, 28
  hormonal changes and, 27
  infections of, 28, 29
  interior of, 30-31, 60-61
  self-examination of, 19, 27-31, 86, 87
  stretch marks on, 31
  surgery for, 27, 137, 138-43
  tenderness of, 83

breath, shortness of, 109
bulbocavernosus muscles, 38
bulb of clitoris, 39, 49, 50

calendar method, in birth control, 105, 106
California, Board of Medical Examiners in
  (BME), 18
California State University at Long Beach,
  "Women and Their Bodies" course at,
  20
CamphoPhenique, 91
cancer, 145
  breast, 109, 138-43
  cervical, 24, 80-81, 92, 109
  ERT and, 76, 77
  uterine, 77, 109
cannula:
  abortion and, 129, 130, 131
  menstrual extraction and, 121, 122,
  125-27
cauterization, types of, 84
CDC (Center for Disease Control), 102
celibacy, 46, 119
Center for Disease Control (CDC), 102
cervical cap, 106, 108, 114-15, 119
  home remedies and, 93
cervicitis, 81, 92
cervix, 92-94
  cancer of, 24, 80-81, 92, 109
  color of, 21, 24, 93, 125
  cysts on, 94
  defined, 22
  difficulties in viewing of, 24, 26
  dilation of, 69, 121, 125, 135
  infections of, 92-93
  os in, 21, 24, 110
  photographing of, 20
  surgery for, 84, 150
  texture of, 21, 24
chemotherapy, 138, 139, 142
chest:
  muscles in, 29
  pain in, 109

chickweed bath, 89
childbirth, 35
 pelvic outlet in, 38
 strengthening muscles for, 40
chills, 100
chlamydia, 93
Cleary, Chris, 34
clitoris, 33-57
 changes in, during sexual excitement, 33-34, 38, 39, 43, 46
 cross sections of, 20, 41, 56-57
 defined, 20, 33-34, 47
 erectile tissue of, 20, 39-40, 49
 manual stimulation of, 35, 47, 50
 muscles of, 20, 38, 40, 41, 52
 outer view of, 34-35, 37, 50, 51
 penis compared to, 46, 48, 49
 secretions of, 39, 62-63
 self-examination of, 33-46
 sexual response cycle and, 48-57
 side view of, 48, 49
cobra exercise, 98
cocoa butter, 31
coffee, 101
coitus:
 function of urethral sponge during, 39, 43
 menopause and, 75
colon, 97
comfrey root, 91
communication:
 as premise of self-help, 17, 21, 87
 between woman and doctor, 79-80
condoms, 106, 108, 115, 119
conization, 150
constipation, 97
Copper-7 IUD, 106, 118
corpus luteum, 71, 72, 73
cramps:
 abortion and, 129, 131, 135
 after cauterization, 84
 IUD and, 106, 117
 in legs, 109
 menstrual, 97-100
 menstrual extraction and, 127
cranberry juice, UTI and, 101
cryosurgery, 84
crypts, 62
cystitis, see urinary tract infections
cysts:
 on breasts, 30, 31, 86, 87, 138, 140
 on cervix, 94

Dalkon Shield, 118
D and C (dilation and curettage), 145-46, 150
D and E (dilation and evacuation), 130, 131
Del-Em, 123-27
Depo-Provera, 119
depression, 76, 77, 97, 109
diaphragms, 18, 105, 106, 108, 112-14, 119
 artificial insemination and, 85
 fitting of, 114
 home remedies and, 92
 menstrual flow and, 102, 103
 removal of, 112, 113
diarrhea, 102
Dickinson, Robert, 34
dilation and curettage (D and C), 145-46, 150
dilation and evacuation (D and E), 130, 131

discharge, 93, 127
 after cauterization, 84
 fibroids and, 97
 vaginal infections and, 22, 82, 89-90
diuretics, 97
doctors:
 breast examinations by, 27
 costs of, 21
 first meeting with, 80
 menstrual extraction and, 121
 techniques for convenience of, 23, 79
 see also medical establishment
donor insemination, 85
douches, douching:
 in birth control, 120
 dangers of, 76
 as home remedy, 89, 90, 93
 sucking air technique for, 90
Downer, Carol, 18, 19, 34
drapes, for medical examinations, 79
dysmenorrhea, 97
dysplasia, 81, 150

Early Pregnancy Test (EPT), 83
E. coli, 89-90
eggs, 66, 67, 71
egg sacs, see follicles
egg tubes, 66, 69, 73, 147
 contraction of, 74
 structure of, 72
endometriosis, 97
endometrium, see uterus, lining of
epilepsy, 77
episiotomies, 35
EPT (Early Pregnancy Test), 83
estrogen-receptor assay (ERA), 139
estrogen replacement therapy (ERT), 76, 77
estrogens, 70, 71
 functions of, 66
examination, well-woman, components of, 78-85
excitement phase, 46, 50, 51
exercise, 21, 76
 pubococcygeal muscle strengthened by, 40
 for relief from cramps, 97-100
experimentation, medical, on women, 19

fallopian tubes, see egg tubes
fatigue, 76, 83, 100
Federation of Feminist Women's Health Centers, 19-20
female ejaculation, 54, 161
feminine deodorants, disadvantages of, 76
feminism, defined, 18
Feminist Women's Health Center (FWHC), 17-19
 establishment of, 17-18
 legal challenge to, 18-19
 see also Federation of Feminist Women's Health Centers
fertile mucus, birth control and, 106, 107, 110-12, 119, 120
fertilization, 105
fever, 100, 102, 127
fibroids, 95-97, 145, 147
flashing lights, sensation of, 109
foam, 115, 119

follicles:
 development of, 71, 72
 primary, 72
 secondary, 72
 tertiary, 72, 73
follicle-stimulating hormone (FSH), 70, 71
forced sterilization, 145
foreplay, see excitement phase
fourchette of clitoris, 34, 35, 37
frenulum, 34, 35, 37
Freud, Sigmund, 34, 46
frigidity, 46
FSH (follicle-stimulating hormone), '70, 71
fundus, 69
FWHC, see Feminist Women's Health Center

Gage, Suzann, 17, 20, 34
Gardnerella vaginalis, 89-90
garlic suppositories, 89, 108
gay. See also lesbians, lesbianism
GC (gonorrhea culture), 84, 85
genital warts, 87-88
glands:
 endocrine, 66, 70-71
 scent, 62-63
 vulvovaginal, 39, 88-89
glans of clitoris, 20, 33, 34, 35, 37, 38
 nerve concentration in, 46
 in self-examination, 36
 sexual response and, 49, 50
glans of penis, 49
goldenseal-root powder, 89, 91, 93
gonorrhea, 92-93, 112
gonorrhea culture (GC), 84, 85
Grafenberg spot, 54
"Great Yogurt Conspiracy, The," 18-19

hair, 66
 around nipples, 28
 pubic, 37
headaches, 97, 109
health-care consumers, women as, 17, 18
Heidelberg, Lynn, 34
Hemophilus, 89-90
hemorrhage, 131, 150
herbal teas, 91, 97
herpes, 90-91
Hirsch, Jeanne and Lolly, 19
Hite, Shere, 47
Hodge, Kathleen, 34
home remedies, 17
 for bladder infections, 101
 douches as, 89
 for dry vagina, 76
 for herpes, 90-91
 limitations of, 84, 87, 93
 for menstrual cramps, 97-100
 for vulvovaginal glands infection, 89
 for yeast condition, 18, 21, 89
homosexual, 159. See also lesbians, lesbianism
honey, 93
hood of clitoris, 20, 33, 35, 37
 sexual response and, 50
hormones:
 breasts affected by, 27
 defined, 71
 functions of, 20, 66, 71
 maturation index of, 82

surgery and, 137
theory of workings of, 71
Hornstein, Francie, 34
hot flashes, 76
Human Sexual Response (Masters and Johnson), 20
Hyde Amendment, 131
hymen, 34, 35, 37
hypoglycemia, 76, 91
hysterectomy, 19, 105, 109, 119, 137, 147
prophylactic, 137
radical, 148-49
simple, 148, 149

infections, 76, 79, 112, 143
breast examination and, 28, 29
in cervical canal, 92-93
menstrual extraction and, 122, 125, 127
symptoms of, 22, 28, 29
urinary tract, 91, 93, 100-101
uterine, 106, 108-9, 127, 131, 145
vaginal, 22, 81, 82, 89-90, 108
venereal, 84
of vulvovaginal glands, 39, 88-89
see also yeast condition
informed consent, right to, 19, 21
insomnia, 76, 83
intestines, 65, 66-67
intimacy, 48
intrauterine devices (IUDs), 116-18, 147
dangers of, 105, 106, 108-9, 121
ischiocavernosus muscles, 38
itching, vaginal, 22, 82
IUDs, *see* intrauterine devices

jaundice, 109
jelly, water-soluble, for speculum insertion, 23
Johnson, Virginia, 20, 33, 34, 46-47

Kegal, Arnold, 40
kidney disease, 77

lactation, 119
Laetrile therapy, 138, 139, 142, 143
laminaria, 131, 134-35
laparoscopy, 144-45
laparotomy, defined, 147
Law, Debra, 19
legs of clitoris, 39
lemon juice, odors removed by, 115
lesbians, lesbianism, 46
health problems of, 84, 87
orgasms of, 47
pregnancy and, 85
liver disease, 76, 77, 91
Los Angeles Women's Center, first FWHC housed in, 18
lumpectomy, 141
lunaception, 106, 120
lysine, 90, 91

mammography, 138-39
massage, 99, 100
mastectomy, 19, 137
modified radical, 142
radical, 138, 139, 143
segmental, 141
simple, 142
Masters, William H., 20, 33, 34, 46-47

masturbation, 47, 76
maturation index, defined, 82
Mead, Margaret, 19
Medicaid, abortion and, 131
medical establishment:
principal focus of, 21
self-help boosted by, 19
self-help *vs.*, 18-19, 21
sexual myths and, 33
menopause, 75-77, 145
sex during, 75
menstrual extraction, 121-27
advantages of, 121
process of, 124-27
risks of, 121, 122, 127
time for, 123
menstruation, menstrual cycle, 66, 71-75, 83
alternatives to tampons and, 102-3
changes in cervix during, 21
cramps during, 97-100
cysts and, 87
hormones in, 71, 72
IUD insertion and, 117
length of, 67
milk glands, 30, 31
miscarriage, 97, 150
induced, 131
Mittelschmerz, 71, 72
moisturizers, for stretch marks, 31
Monthly Extract, 19
Morales, Sylvia, 20
Morgan, Robin, 19
muscles, 66
of clitoris, 20, 38, 40, 41, 52
pelvic, 52
relaxation of, 97-100
myomectomy, 97
myrrh, 89, 91

National Abortion Federation, 19
National Organization for Women (NOW), 18
National Women's Studies Association, 20
Nature and Evolution of Female Sexuality, The (Sherfey), 34
nausea, 83
neosporin ointment, 91
nerves, of clitoris, 20, 34, 46
New Zealand, self-help in, 19
nipples, 29, 141
inverted, 28
squeezing of, 28
NOW (National Organization for Women), 18
nursing, stretch marks from, 31
nutrition, 21, 76
herpes and, 90-91
menstrual cycle and, 67

orgasm, 17, 34, 46-49, 52
age and first experience of, 48
clitoral muscle in, 38, 52
cramps and, 97
vaginal, 33, 46, 47
orgasmic platform, 34
os, defined, 21, 24
Our Bodies, Ourselves, 20
ovaries, 71-73
atrophy of, 76, 77
defined, 71
hormones produced by, 66, 70

removal of, 71, 139
sexual response and, 50
ovulation, 67, 71, 72, 73, 74
fertile mucus and, 111-12
fertilization and, 105
after menopause, 76
temperature change and, 106, 107

pants, tight-fitting, problems caused by, 76, 87
paraurethral ducts, 43, 161
Pap smears, 19, 24, 80-82, 92
classifying results of, 81
method used in, 80, 81
patient advocate, role of, 21, 80
patient's rights, 19, 21
summary of, 80
pelvic bones, 42, 65
pelvic diaphragm, 40
pelvic inflammatory disease, 93
pelvic muscles, in orgasm phase, 52
pelvic outlet, 38
penis, 43
clitoris compared to, 46, 48, 49
cross sections of, 33
peppermint tea, 91
perineal sponge, 39, 40
self-examination of, 45
sexual response and, 50
perineum, 37, 38
Pill, the
bleeding and, 105-6
cysts and, 87
dangers of, 105-6, 109, 121
delayed menstruation after discontinuation of, 67, 105
ERT compared to, 77
infections and, 93
pituitary glands, 70
plateau phase, 46, 50, 51
podophyllum, 88
polyps, 95
Ponstel, 97
population control, 161
pregnancy:
artificial insemination and, 85
classic signs of, 83
drug use during, 91
fibroids and, 97
menstrual extraction and, 122, 125, 127
stretch marks from, 31
testing for, 83, 129
progestogens, 70, 71, 72
functions of, 66
prostaglandins, 97
providone-iodine, 91
pubic bone, 38, 39, 52
pubococcygeal muscle, 40
pyridium, 91

racism, 145, 161
radiation therapy, 138, 139, 142
rashes, 52, 102
rectovaginal exam, 79
rectum, 40, 52
relaxation techniques, 97-100
resolution phase, 53
respect, as health-care right, 19
rhythm method, in birth control, 105, 106
Right-to-Life movement, 131
Rothman, Lorraine, 19, 34, 123

sanitary napkins, 102
Schiffer, Sherry, 34
sea sponges, menstrual flow and, 102, 103
self-examination, 21-31
    benefits of, 22, 27
    of breasts, 19, 27-31, 86, 87
    of cervix, 19, 21, 22-26
    of clitoris, 33-46
    image improved by, 18
    legal challenge to, 18-19
    sexism as obstacle to, 17
    tools for, 21
    of uterus, 68-69
    of vagina, 19, 22-26
self-help:
    cost factors in, 17, 21, 102, 123
    feminism as basis of, 18
    grass roots of, 17-20
    Iowa conference on (1972), 19
    national audience created for, 18-19, 21
    research for, 19-20
    self-care movement distinguished from,
        21
self-help clinics, 17-20, 153-54
    conceptual basis of, 17
    first, 17-18
semen, 85, 115
sexism, in need for self-help, 17
sexual response, 46-57
    cycle of, 48-57
    excitement phase of, 46, 50, 51
    function of urethral sponge in, 39, 43
    myths about, 33, 46-47
    orgasm phase of, 46, 52
    plateau phase of, 46, 50, 51
    resolution phase of, 53
    restrictions on, 47
shaft of clitoris, 20, 33, 34, 35, 38, 39
    in self-examination, 36
    sexual response and, 49, 50
    stimulation of, 35
shaft of penis, 49
Sherfey, Mary Jane, 34
Shiatsu, 100
Sitz baths, 89, 91
skin, 31, 66
smoking, 76
speculums, 21-26, 89
    defined, 21
    doctor's conventional use of, 23
    insertion of, 22-23
    in menstrual extraction, 124, 125
    purchasing of, 21, 23
    types of, 25-26
sperm, 71, 105, 110-11
spermicides, 108, 112, 115, 119
squamocolumnar junction, 92
Staph bacteria, 89-90, 102
Steinem, Gloria, 19
sterility, 85
sterilization, 19, 119, 144-45, 151
    abuse, 145, 162
stimulants, 91, 101
stirrups, putting feet in, 23, 79
Stoxil, 91
strep, 89-90

stress:
    herpes and, 90, 91
    menstrual cycle and, 67
stretch marks, on breasts, 31
strokes, 109
sucking air technique, 90
sulfa cream, 91
suppositories, 89, 108, 120
Supreme Court, U.S., abortion rulings by,
    19, 121, 129, 131
surgery, 87, 97, 136-51
    alternatives to, 138, 139, 143
    breast, 27, 137, 138-43
    for cervical infection, 84, 150
    disfiguration due to, 19, 137, 143
    trauma of, 138
    unnecessary, 19, 137
    see also specific procedures
symptothermic method, in birth control,
    106, 119

tampons, 89, 102, 103
thermography, 138-39
thyroid problems, 76
toxic shock syndrome (TSS), 102
tranquilizers, 76
transverse perineal muscles, 38
trichomonas, 22
    symptoms of, 82, 89
    testing for, 81, 82
    treatment for, 89, 90
TSS (toxic shock syndrome), 102
tubal ligation, 119, 144-45
2-deoxy d-glucose (2-DDG), 91

urethra, 34, 35, 37, 40, 52
    protection of, 39, 43
urethral sponge, 39, 40, 43
    self-examination of, 44
    sexual response and, 50
urinary tract infections (UTI), 91, 93,
    100-101
urination:
    frequency of, 83, 100
    painful, 91, 100
urine pregnancy test, 83
uterus, 38, 64-69
    cancer of, 77, 109
    contractions of, 97
    fibroid tumors on, 95-97
    infections of, 106, 108-9, 127, 131, 145
    ligaments as support for, 67, 72
    lining of, 62, 66, 69, 74-75
    midline, 68, 69
    perforation of, 130, 150
    relaxation of, 97-100
    self-examination of, 68-69
    sexual response and, 50, 55, 69
    size check of, 78, 79, 95, 96-97
    tipped, 68, 69, 79
UTI (urinary tract infections), 91, 93,
    100-101

vagina, 40
    clitoral opening to, 34, 35, 37
    dry, 76

infections of, 22, 81, 82, 89-90, 108
    orgasm and, 33, 46, 47
    orgasmic platform in, 34
    secretions of, 21, 22, 50, 62-63, 76, 82
    self-examination of, 19, 22-26
    sexual response and, 50, 53, 55
vaginal creams, yogurt vs., 21
vaginitis, nonspecific, 89-90
vasectomy, 119, 151
vasocongestion, defined, 50
venereal disease, testing for, 84
venereal warts, 87-88
vinegar:
    douche, 90
    odors removed by, 102, 115'
vitamins, 76, 93
    cancer and, 138, 139, 142, 143
    herpes prevention and, 90-91
    hormones and, 71
    stretch marks and, 31
vomiting, 102
vulva:
    defined, 37
    inner lips of, 34-35
    outer lips of, 33, 34, 35, 37
    secretions of, 62-63
vulvovaginal glands, infection of, 39, 88-89

Walker, Lynn, 34
Walker, Nancy, 34
water:
    retention of, 97, 109
    UTI and, 101
weight changes:
    in menopause, 76
    Pill and, 109
    stretch marks due to, 31
white body, 72
Wilson, Colleen, 18
withdrawal, 120
Women's Health in Women's Hands, 19-20
Women's Health Movement, 19, 102
women's health projects:
    addresses of, 164-67
    as source of speculums, 23
Women's Liberation Movement, self-help
    as part of, 18, 19

xeroradiography, 138-39
X-rays, 116, 138-39
Xylocaine jelly, 91

yarrow tea, 97
yeast condition:
    causes of, 89, 101
    symptoms of, 82, 89
    testing for, 81, 82
    treatment for, 18, 21, 89
yellow body, see corpus luteum
yogurt:
    dry vagina treated with, 76
    insertion method for, 89
    yeast condition treated with, 18, 21, 89

zinc oxide, 91

ABOUT THE AUTHORS

In 1975, three woman-owned, woman controlled health centers located in Los Angeles and Orange County, California, and in Tallahassee, Florida, formed the Federation of Feminist Women's Health Centers to increase their impact within the Women's Health Movement and to work very closely on projects of common concern.

The federation now consists of health centers in Chico, Redding, Sacramento and Santa Rosa, California, Atlanta, Georgia, Eugene and Portland, Oregon, and Renton and Yakima Washington. An associate member clinic is in Tallahassee Florida.

Women from the federation actively participate in national organizations like the American Public Health Association, the National Abortion Federation, the National Organization for Women and the National Women's Studies Association. Federation members participate in a number of progressive community groups and work with many women's rights organizations. Although the health centers work closely on many projects, each has it's own particular character and relationship to the community.

The Los Angeles Feminist Women's Health Center, no longer in existence, was the first to be established, in 1972. Although this book was a federation project over a period of five years, the writing and research were done largely in Los Angeles. In addition to working on the book, individual women on the staff had positions in the area of women's health outside of the health center. Ginny Cassidy-Brinn was Vice President of the California Board of Registered Nursing, and Gail Goldstein coordinated a course called "Women and Their Bodies," which was team taught by the health center staff at California State University at Long Beach. Carol Downer was secretary and on the Executive Committee of the National Abortion Federation, and France Hornstein, was on the Executive Committee of the National Women's Health Network.

The Chico Feminist Women's Health Center is the only abortion clinic in rural Norther California. Dido Hasper, a founder of the Chico Health Center, has been a coordinator of the federation, and the Chico staff does much of the federations legislative work on women's health issues on the state level in nearby Sacramento.

The Orange County Feminist Women's Health Center, located in Santa Ana, also no longer in existence, was the first abortion facility in Orange County. In 1979 the staff initiated an innovative program at Chapman College in Orange to maintain a clinic annex on the campus to provide pregnancy screening, a participatory well-woman clinic and self-help clinics.

Womancare, A Feminist Women's Health Center, in San Diego, initiated the only woman-controlled birth program of it's type in 1973 Through this program, women received prenatal care at the clinic and then had the option of a home or hospital birth attended by the center's physician. The program ended when pressure from the local medical society caused Womancare's physicians to be unwilling to attend home births. Clinic staff conducted a survey of birth conditions across the United States.

The Feminist Women's Health Center in Atlanta is one of three woman-controlled clinics in the South. The health center has worked diligently to try to keep Medicaid funds available for abortions for poor women and to ensure that new state clinic regulations would not restrict abortion.

Everywoman's Clinic, A Feminist Women's Health Center, in Pleasant Hill, California, also no longer in existence, was often the target of local anti-abortion groups. but with the support of women's groups and individual women in the community, it was successful in keeping high-quality abortion care available.

Although this book is the result of the collective efforts of more than one hundred women, some women were delegate the primary responsibility for illustrations, photography and writing.

SUZANN GAGE, L Ac, RNC,NP, is founder and executive director of Wholistic Health for Women and the Lesbian Health Clinic in Los Angeles, California, and is a licensed acupuncturist and certified nurse practitioner. While a director of the Los Angeles Feminist Women's Health Center she authored *When Birth Control Fails*, coauthored and illustrated *How To Stay Out of the Gynecologists Office*, and illustrated *Woman Centered Pregnancy and Birth*, and *The Hit Report on Male Sexuality*. She also illustrated *The Complete Cervical Cap Guide*, and *Overcoming Bladder Disorders*.

SYLVIA MORALES, after making *A New Image of Myself*, a film about self-examination in 1975, participated in a cross country tour to do the photographs for this book. Her documentary on the history of Chicana-Mexican women from pre-Columbian times to the present, entitled *Chicana*, was released in 1979 and has been widely distributed. She currently has her own independent film company called Sylvan Productions in Los Angeles.

CAROL DOWNER, JD, Is founding director of the Federation of Feminist Women's Health Centers, and was founder and executive director of the Feminist Women's Health Center in Los Angeles. She both supervised and directly participated in the editing of this text. which is based on research and concepts that she and other women from the health centers formulate. She is currently a civil rights attorney in Los Angeles and is coauthor of *How To Stay Out of the Gynecologist's Office, Woman Centered Pregnancy and Birth,* and *A Woman's Book Of Choices.*

REBECCA CHALKER, MA, a freelance writer in New York City who holds a master's degree in English from Florida State University, edited the current text from a larger work of 350,000 words. She is author of *The Complete Cervical Cap Guide,* and coauthor of *Overcoming Bladder Disorders*, and *A Woman's Book of Choices*. She is a partner in Womancap, New York City's most active cervical cap provider.

SANDRA SULLAWAY GIBBINGS, a founder of the Women's Community Health Center in Cambridge, Massachusetts, coordinated the technical aspects of the first printing of the book. She is on the board of directors of the Women's Fund, and is active in La Leche League. She currently lives in Michigan and is the mother of two sons.

Celebrating Women's Health!
A New View of a Woman's Body

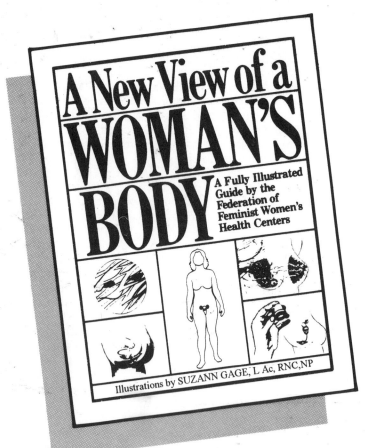

A New View of a WOMAN'S BODY

A Fully Illustrated Guide by the Federation of Feminist Women's Health Centers

Illustrations by SUZANN GAGE, L Ac, RNC,NP

In true celebration of women's health, *A New View of a Woman's Body* is available now in paper back from Feminist Health Press.

First published in 1981 by Simon and Schuster, this exquisitely illustrated and photographed book was lovingly written by the Federation of Feminist Women's Health Centers to demystify women's bodies and health care, and to empower women with vaginal self-examination and other self-help techniques.

Based on ten years of self-help research, *A New View of a Woman's Body* presents clear, detailed descriptions of vaginal and breast self-examination, the anatomy of the clitoris, common infections, lab tests, birth control, menstrual extraction, abortion care, menopause, surgical procedures, and home remedies.

A perfect companion to *Our Bodies Ourselves*!

Available in bookstores. To order:
